D0049820

Art and Aesthetics in Nursing

Art and Aesthetics in Nursing

Peggy L. Chinn and Jean Watson, Editors

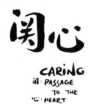

关心

CARING
闰 PASSAGE
TO THE
'心' HEART

Center for Human Caring

National League for Nursing Press • *New York*
Pub. No. 14-2611

Copyright © 1994
National League for Nursing
350 Hudson Street, New York, NY 10014

ISBN 0-88737-609-6

This book was set in Garamond by Publications Development of Texas. The ed-
itor and designer was Allan Graubard with Maryan Malone. Northeastern Press
was the printer and binder.

The cover was designed by Lauren Stevens.

Printed in the United States of America

Contents

Contributors

Cathy Appleton, PhD, ARNP, CS
Interim Graduate Program Director
College of Nursing
Florida Atlantic University
Boca Raton, FL

Jennifer B. Averill, MSN, RN
Instructor and PhD student
University of Colorado
School of Nursing
Denver, CO

D. Ellen Boyle, MS, RN
Clinical Nurse Specialist
Children's Hospital
Seattle, WA

Karen Breunig, RN
University of Colorado
School of Nursing
Denver, CO

Elizabeth R. Bruderle, MSN, RN
College of Nursing
Villanova University
Villanova, PA

Patricia M. Casey, MSN, BSN
Neonatal Nurse Practitioner
Denver, CO

Peggy L. Chinn, PhD, RN, FAAN
Professor of Nursing
Associate Dean for Academics
University of Colorado Health Sciences Center
Denver, CO

Sharon Ann Cumbie, RN, MS
Doctoral student
University of Colorado Health Sciences Center
Denver, CO

Mary Koithan, PhD, RN
University of Colorado Health Sciences Center
Instructor of Nursing
University of Nevada, Las Vegas

Suzanne Kusserow, EdD, RNC
1994 Fulbright Scholar to Zimbabwe
Mary T. Rockwood Lane
Center of the Healing Arts
Shands Hospital
Gainesville, FL

Mary Hobbs Leenerts, RN, MS
PhD student
University of Colorado
School of Nursing
Denver, CO

M. Katherine Maeve, MS, RN
Doctoral candidate, Nursing
University of Colorado Health Sciences Center
HIV Early Intervention Clinical Nurse Specialist
Denver Health and Hospitals
Denver, CO

Judy Malkiewicz, PhD, RN
Associate Professor of Nursing
University of Northern Colorado
Greeley, CO

Shirley A. Mealey, PhD, RN
University of Colorado
School of Nursing
Denver, CO

Wanda K. Mohr, PhD candidate, MA, RN
University of Texas at Austin

John Graham Pole

Mary T. Rockwood, PhD candidate, MA, BS
University of Florida
College of Nursing
Gainsville, FL

Sarah R. Rutherfoord

Marilyn L. Stember, PhD, RN, FAAN
Professor of Nursing
Associate Dean for Research
University of Colorado Health Sciences Center
Denver, CO

Joanne Marky Supples, PhD, RN
Assistant Professor, Nursing
University of Colorado
School of Nursing
Denver, CO

Phyllis A. Updike, PhD, RN
Assistant Professor, Nursing
University of Colorado
School of Nursing
Denver, CO

Theresa M. Valiga, EdD, RN
College of Nursing
Villanova University
Villanova, PA

Toni M. Vezeau, PhD, RN
Assistant Clinical Professor
University of Colorado Health Sciences Center
Maternal-Child Clinician
University Hospital
Denver, CO

Jean Watson, PhD, RN, FAAN
Distinguished Professor of Nursing
Director, Center for Human Caring
University of Colorado Health Sciences Center
Denver, CO

Introduction: Art and Aesthetics as Passage between Centuries

The most beautiful experience we can have is the mysterious . . . the fundamental emotion which stands at the cradle of true art and true science.

Albert Einstein (1879-1955)

As the twentieth century ends, nursing stands poised between the past and the future. Epochal changes have taken place and are predicted in the caring-healing arts. Yet, as Donahue (1985) says, many of the extraordinary innovations that have occurred are continuations of contributions from the past; they have resulted from a new integration and linkage of the past and the present. Within this century, health care services have moved from health spas and herbal natural healing centers to penthouses, to comprehensive, technologically sophisticated medical treatment settings, and toward a new reintegration of mind/body/soul and environment with the art and aesthetics of caring and healing.

During the past two decades, nursing has advanced by critiquing existing epistemologies, questioning ethical perspectives, and witnessing and experiencing the dominance of technology and the functional tasks of medical treatment.

> *[T]he real essence of nursing, as of any fine art, lies not in the mechanical details of execution, nor yet in the dexterity of the performer, but in the creative imagination, the sensitive spirit, and the intelligent understanding lying back of these techniques and skills. Without these, nursing may become a highly skilled trade, but it cannot be a profession or a fine art. (Stewart, 1929/1985)*

As leaders in many fields have pointed out, all the rituals and ceremonials that our modern worship of efficiency may devise, and all our elaborate scientific equipment, will not save the art of nursing if its intellectual and spiritual elements are subordinated to its mechanical elements and if the *means* at our disposal are regarded as more important than the *ends* for which they were devised.

In the past decade, the history of nursing, portrayed through art, has demonstrated the most valuable aspect of nursing: care and caring. However, no one, through pen or canvas, will ever be able to entirely capture the true art and the caring spirit of nursing. As Donahue (1985) reminded us, they both defy expression.

Nursing has faithfully transmitted its skills from one generation and from one century to the next. But as we are poised to begin the twenty-first century, . . . a new transmission is under way: art that has been buried from the public eye of nursing and science is being readied to become visible. Nurses dwell in the human realm, and within that realm art sustains our dual human and spirit life. Through art, we are able to reconnect with and remember our lost knowledge, to bridge the erosions and exclusions that nursing's consciousness was subject to during this century (Smith, 1982). The lost art of nursing is now being reclaimed and restored.

"Nursing is an art," wrote Nightingale (1859/1992), "and if it is to be made an art, it requires as exclusive a devotion, as hard a preparation, as any painter's or sculptor's work."

Her words place nursing, the oldest art, among the fine arts. Her ringing tribute to the human spirit, "What's dead canvas and cold marble compared with the living body, the temple of God's spirit?", reminds us that the art of nursing deals with the human spirit and that "Nursing activities are the art from which patients are enabled to spiritually develop."

Parker (1988) referred to art as a medium for forming or deforming the human soul, the life spirit. Art captures, expresses, and recreates humanity and life in all their various and diverse forms. Art evokes spirituality, inspiration, imagination, creativity, and dedication. Art is the life's spirit.

Of art and the spirit, Emerson (1982) said: "Nature is the symbol of the spirit, nature always wears the colors of the spirit; art conspires with the spirit in search of beauty, wisdom, truth" (p. 48). Truth, as defined by Keats (1819/1993), "Beauty is "Truth, Truth beauty . . . ," is not scientific truth, more easily pursued and captured, but inner, more elusive, universal truth flowing from nature and life itself.

Art conspires with the spirit to emancipate us; art allows us to locate ourselves in another space and place, to change our perceptions, our points of view. The relations of the parts and the whole shift; art and nature alike apprehend the unity of nature, which is a unity in variety. When nursing is properly identified as a fine art, these words of Emerson (1982) are exhilarating:

The production of a work of art throws a light upon the mystery of humanity. A work of art is an abstract or epitome of the world. It is the result or expression of Nature in miniature. Thus in art does Nature work through [a human will] filled with the beauty of her first works. . . . The world thus exits to the soul to satisfy the desire of beauty. This element I call an ultimate end. No reason can be asked or given why the soul seeks beauty. Beauty, in its largest and profoundest sense, is an expression for the universe. (pp. 47, 48)

Emerson also reminds us of the deep connection among beauty, art, and the soul of humanity. The soul has been identified as the very font of who we are, yet the concept of *soul* goes beyond who we are and exceeds our capacity to devise and control; we can't outwit it or manage it. "Art and soul are linked through the sacred nature of both" (Moore, 1992).

The art of nursing is the capacity of a human being to receive another human being's expression of feelings and to experience those feelings for oneself. The artistic expression of nursing includes intentional auditory, visual, sensory, olfactory, and tactile art or acts (Updike, 1992). Among these are purposive movement, touch, sound, color, form, nature, and so on. Nursing as art is lived, expressed, and cocreated in the caring moment. (Watson, 1988). Gendron (1988) suggested that the aesthetic character of the expressive form of caring, as revealed in the perception and action of the nurse, includes direction, force, balance, and rhythm.

In nursing in the twentieth century, spirituality was separated from art, and art was separated from science. Nursing must be radically reimagined if it is to restore its caring–healing fine art and the view of mind/body/spirit unity that is the basis of its practice. In this revision, nursing art and spirituality—the sacred—need to be seen again as one.

This reintegrating paradigm of caring–healing arts suggests the end of modern nursing as we have known it. New visions, new vocabulary, and new traditions are being developed that reach back into our distant past and look toward greater fulfillment in our future.

This anthology of art and aesthetics in nursing emerged from our awareness of a growing scholarly interest in the art of nursing and the aesthetic pattern of knowing in nursing. Unsure whether the level of interest evident at the University of Colorado was shared by scholars elsewhere, we placed a call for papers, not wholly confident of the response we would receive. The chapters contained herein represent only half of the manuscripts we received and reviewed.

The themes that emerged are represented by the four Parts of the anthology:

I.   Art as Asking and Knowing.
II. Art as Learning.
III. Art as Practice.
IV. Art as Reflective Experience.

The chapter groupings are not meant to fully define each of these themes; rather, they illustrate possibilities in our collective and growing awareness of the art of nursing and aesthetic knowing in nursing.

The introduction of this anthology of art and aesthetics in nursing as the year 2000 approaches seems highly appropriate. At this juncture in nursing's history, it is time to take back what has been disowned; to reclaim, celebrate, and give testimony to the art of nursing; and to do so with a devotion that pleases the soul. We invite our readers to drink it up and enjoy its refreshment.

M. JEAN WATSON AND PEGGY L. CHINN

Denver, Colorado
April 1994

REFERENCES

Donahue, P. (1985). *Nursing: The finest art.* St. Louis: Mosby.

Emerson, R. W. (1982). *Selected essays.* Middlesex, England: Penguin Books.

Gendron, D. (1988). *The expressive form of caring.* Toronto, Canada: University of Toronto.

Keats, J. (1993). Ode on a Grecian urn (1819). In *Norton anthology of poems* (p. 664). New York: Norton.

Moore, T. (1992). *Care of the soul.* New York: HarperCollins.

Nightingale, F. (1859). *Notes on nursing.* London: Harrison and Sons. (Commemorative Edition. (1992). Philadelphia: Lippincott.)

Parker, P. (1987). Community, conflict, and ways of knowing. *The Magazine of Higher Learning, 19*(5), 20-25.

Smith, H. (1982). *Beyond the postmodern mind.* New York: Crossroad Publishing. (Reissued. (1984). Wheaton, IL: Theosophical Publishing.)

Stewart, I. (1985). In P. Donahue, *Nursing: The finest art* (p. 467). St. Louis: Mosby. (Original work published 1929)

Updike, P. (1992). Personal communication, University of Colorado Center for Human Caring, Denver.

Watson, J. (1988). *Nursing: Human science, human care.* New York: National League for Nursing.

Part I

Art as Asking and Knowing

Poeticizing as Truth through Language

Jean Watson

"What is Truth?" A question asked down through the ages. And what does poetry have to do with Truth? We are well aware that poetry has a place in the life of the mind, of imagination, of evocation, and we may eventually consider poetry as a way or a form of knowing. But what could its relation be to that most fundamental pursuit—the search for Truth—and to Truth itself?

We must not interfere with that relation, even if we enjoy our own experience with poetry. The pursuit of Truth is beyond question in the world of science. Is poetry then better placed outside the world of Truth and science?

I suppose our present, separatist ontology of knowing, with respect to Western world science, would have us take that position. Guba and Lincoln (1989) gave this definition of the conventional nature of truth: "The truth of any proposition (its factual quality) can be determined by testing it empirically in the natural world. Any proposition that has withstood such a test is True; such Truth is absolute" (p. 104). Within this conditioned perspective, Truth is defined as a result of an appropriate inquiry or methodology—namely, the experiment conducted in a value-free context—leading to a ritual of method. Nietzsche captured this dilemma precisely: "It is not the victory of science that distinguishes this century, but the victory of scientific method over science" (Gadamer, 1988, p. xii). However, as we search for Truth, we do not, nor cannot, stand outside the world of method of truthmaking. Even phenomenology, as a liberating model for human science, was originally understood within science, reflecting a tendency that has essentially meant the dominance of method (Gadamer, 1988).

Indeed, in Gadamer's (1991) *Truth and Method,* he sought to show the drawbacks of methodology's rule within the human sciences. In doing so, he turned to the arts and poetry to gain access to a truth more irresistible than that offered by the sometimes dogmatic applications of method. As Palmer Parker (1987) recently reminded us, we must be careful with our development of knowledge and Truth because "we shape souls by the nature of our knowledge." As we now understand, Truth is not necessarily discovered *without,* but by interplay and interpretation.

Because we are humans, our Truths are cocreated through a process of values and meaning-making via language. When those values become human values of caring for self, others, and all living things, including planet Earth, and when the meaning-making of Truth involves humans and cocreation of meaning via language, then another scenario, different from the one we are used to, reveals the possibility of poeticizing as Truth. Poets often lie to get at Truth, but their language is haunting and will not be silenced because poetry is the language of people. As Gadamer (1991) explains, the current ontological shift toward hermeneutics is guided by language: language as experience of the world and language as horizon of a hermeneutic ontology, reminding us again that Truth is not necessarily discovered *without* but by interpretation and meaning.

This scenario of Truth via language, meaning, and experience involves our ability to choose among ways of knowing, being, and doing. We do not have the option of not seeking Truth, of "not knowing, because it is the nature of beings like us with subjectivity to use language to formulate meanings" (Gadow, 1990, p. 2), to come to some Truth within our world and ourselves.

Both Merleau Ponty (1962) and Heidegger (1971, 1977) were clear on this point. The former explained that we are given to ourselves as something to be understood, and the latter pointed to being itself: our being hears the call of a language that speaks to the being of all things that respond, a mortal language that speaks of what it hears. Thus, because knowing through language and Truth seeking are part of our being, we cannot decline this process. But we can decide whether the Truth we seek shall be a means of refusing life (what Heidegger called concealment) or of disengaging from life and gaining for ourselves a distance from the world (Gadow, 1990). If we seek or accept such distance by strategies of disengagement and concealment, thereby preserving an object-stance relationship with the world, then we have opted for a model of Truth and knowing that science for centuries has called its own (Gadow, 1990). Such Truth making requires a theory based on traditional, causal relationships between facts and the physical universe. Causality, however, does not bear sufficient witness to the complexity of phenomena characteristic of life. Again, its language is one of concealment. Given such language, values (both subjective and imaginative) that evoke multiple contexts of meanings and of our "authentic relations as mortal to other mortals, to earth, and sky, to the divinities present or absent, to things and plants and animals" (Hofstadter, 1975) remain hidden. Perhaps equally important here is the acceptance we too easily grant to eliminating any correspondence between Beauty and Truth. This correspondence, as it unfolds, returns us to Keats (1983), when he wrote in *Ode on a Grecian Urn:*

Beauty is Truth,
Truth beauty—that is
all ye know on earth,
and all ye need to know. *(p. 664)*

If we can identify with Keats and with poetry as a form of Truth and beauty, we can rejoin the world as inhabitants, open to our being and to the being of others, via human language and aesthetics. If we can cross over into the world of authentic being and hold ourselves open, then we can experience and reside in both outer Truth and inner, self-evident Truth. We shall be authentic residents, not aliens who are separate and separated from our own Truth, so much disclaimed by disengaged, causal models of Truth.

Within Keats's view of Truth, poetry presides. Its task is "to instruct as well as to please." Poetry is thus valid in both classical aesthetics and contemporary science, at least within a human science model that elicits a more vivacious, reflected, and reflective form of Truth as coconstituted in a mortal language that speaks of what we hear and experience.

In Heidegger's (1971) view, the speech of genuine thinking is by nature *poetic*. Nor need it take the shape of verse; this is not a matter of form. In this sense, the opposite of poetry is not prose; pure prose is as poetic as any poetry.

> *[T]he voice of thought must be poetic because poetry is the saying of Truth, the saying of the unconcealedness of beings. . . . Poetry that thinks is in truth the topology of being. This topology tells Being the whereabouts of its actual presence. (p. 12)*

According to Gadamer (1988), the art of language decides not only the success or failure of poetry, but also its claim to Truth. The Platonic objection to the trustworthiness of poetry and poets—"Poets often lie"—opposes the belief in the truthfulness of art generally, and this claim still is not easily silenced (p. 106).

But Heidegger (1971, 1977) indicated that we have a slight and stunted knowledge of the nature of Truth, as evidenced by the laxity we permit ourselves in using this basic word. Truth means usually this or that particular truth: *something* true. But what does "in truth" mean: is it the same or different? For Heidegger, "in truth" referred to the essence of the true; those features held in common by everything that is true, in the generic and universal concept.

In this way, the nature of Truth is found, as it was for Keats, in the Greek *Aletheia,* which Heidegger (1971) interpreted as the unconcealment of beings (pp. 50-51). This unconcealment occurs in life, in the midst of beings, in an open space, a clearing that is created and never set, never concluded. But as the clearing opens up, it also conceals. It carries its negation in its own unfolding. It is never merely an existent state. Thus, we begin to see that unconcealment (via Truth, for Heidegger) is never reduced to sheer factual things, because the unfolding of facts expresses the ambiguities of meaning and of being.

Truth also carries its own negation: "Truth in its nature is untruth" (Heidegger, 1971, p. 54). Yet this does not mean that truth is falsehood nor does it mean that truth is never itself. Truth *is* viewed dialectically—it is also its opposite.

Within these ambiguities, perhaps we can now ask: How does Truth happen? Heidegger put it this way: Truth happens when that

Vincent Van Gogh, "Three Pairs of Shoes," 1887. Oil on canvas, 18" × 28½". Courtesy of the Fogg Art Museum, Harvard University. Bequest—Collection of Maurice Wertheim, Class of 1906.

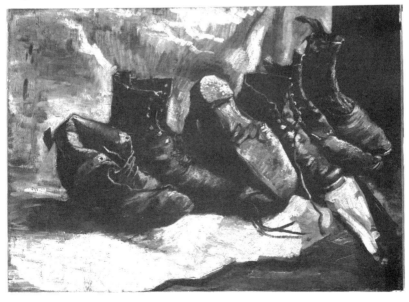

which is as a whole is brought into unconcealment and held therein, meaning further "to hold, to keep, to take care of." To illustrate, Heidegger (1971) turned to a painting by Van Gogh, "Three Pairs of Shoes." In the painting, Truth "does not mean everything is correctly portrayed, but rather that in the revelation of the being of the shoes, that which is as a whole—world and earth in their counterplay—attains to unconcealedness" (p. 56).

As Truth is in art, so it is in poetry. To convey an image, a poem tells of a "*Roman* fountain"; another says "so much depends/upon/ a red wheel/barrow/glazed with rain/water/beside the white/ chickens" (W. C. Williams, 1923/1983, p. 945). Their purpose is not to:

> *just make manifest anything at all; rather, they make un-concealedness as such happen to regard to what is as a whole. The more simply and authentically the items are engrossed in their nature, the more directly and engagingly do all beings attain to a greater degree of being along with them. . . . That is how self-concealing being is illuminated. Light of this kind joins its shining to and into the work. This shining, joined in the work, is the beautiful. Beauty is one way in which Truth occurs as unconcealedness. (Heidegger, 1971, p. 56)*

Thus, we return to William Carlos Williams' *red wheel/barrow* and to Heidegger's position that the nature of Truth is as much the unconcealment of beings as it is the nature of being.

With this inversion of the closed world of Truth, in which we conceal and are cut off from our world, we recover a world of Truth in poeticizing—things are opened up, unfolded to us in a world far too inexhaustible to be seen as closed or limited. Gadow (1990) cautioned, "[T]here is no getting to the end of it because we know it [now through language of poetry] from within, not from outside" (p. 14).

In this world that we can know from the inside, through language and poetry, there can be no falseness; there is no external standard against which Truth can be measured and to which

Truth might correspond. Yet, this world is far from arbitrary. It represents a unique kind of risk because it can fail to live up to itself. In poetry, this Truth happens not because it fails to correspond to "facts," but because its work proves to be "empty." According to Gadamer (1988), this occurs when, instead of sounding "right," it merely sounds like other poetry or like the rhetoric of everyday life. When the work fulfills itself and becomes language, revealing to us a human depth otherwise overlooked, we must take it at its word.

Another feature of poetry as Truth we must consider as purely poetic; that is, poetry is not fulfilled by anything beyond itself or by any confirmation we might seek through verification of facts or further experience. "Poetry fulfills itself" (Gadamer, 1988, p. 111). Or, in Heidegger's terms: "Poetically man Dwells" (Hofstadter, 1975).

At the same time that poetry fulfills itself and we dwell therein as our being, poetry evokes an image and an idea of something beyond, for example, the literal "fountain" or "wheel barrow." We do not look in the direction of any particular fountain or wheel barrow, but each of us constructs an image of a "Roman fountain" or "red wheel barrow." We construct the world of the poem from within the poem itself, and it provokes an immediate refusal to seek verification for what is said, heard, or read. It fulfills itself.

Gadamer (1988, p. 111) explained why we do not sense (in contrast with the casual, scientific, empirical verification model) a need for verification here. A genuine poem allows us to experience "nearness" in and through the linguistic form of the poem. In other words, although fundamental human experiences always change and are constantly subject to change, "the poem does not fade, for the poetic word brings the transience of time to a standstill . . ." It stands written, where its own presence is in play. Gadamer (1988) also stated that this standing of the work is related to the fundamental situation initially described by Hegel as "feeling at home in the world" (p. 114).

For Gadamer (1988), the poem not only helps us in "making ourselves at home," but also stands at the side, holding up our familiarity to us as in a mirror:

But what appears in this mirror is not the world, nor this or that thing in the world, but rather, this nearness or familiarity itself in which we stand for a while. . . . this is but a description of the fact that language gives all of us our access to a world in which certain special forms of human experience arise; . . . the poetic word that by being there bears witness to our own being. (p. 115)

POETRY AS METHOD OF TRUTH: UNCONCEALMENT THROUGH LANGUAGE FROM THE INSIDE OUT

Marilyn Krysl's (1989) poetry about caring and nursing informs us, from the inside out, about the unconcealment of language. She helps us see how we dwell poetically within the most seemingly mundane acts that turn toward keeping alive the human condition, the human spirit, through the interior dimensions of our art—our acts of being with and for another.

Consider Krysl's (1989) description of a nurse and patient who enter into each other's world and dwell poetically therein through the poetry itself, which provides its own "Truth" to the experience:

Sunshine Acres Living Center

The first thing you see up ahead is Mr.
Polanski, wedged in the
arched doorway, like he means absolutely
to stay there, he who shouldn't
be here in the first place, put in here by mistake, courtesy
*   of that grandson*
who thinks himself a hotshot, and too busy
raking in the dough to find time for an old
man. If Polanski had anyplace
to go, he'd be out
instantly, if he had any
money. Which he doesn't, but he does have
a sharp eye, and intends to stay in that

doorway, not missing a thing, and waiting
for trouble. Which of course
will come. And could be
you—you're handy, you look
likely, you have

the authority. And
you're new here, another young
whippersnapper, doesn't know
ass from elbow, but has been give
the keys. Well he's

ready, Polanski. Mr. Polanski, good
morning—*you say it in Polish,*
which you learned a little of
when you were little, and your grandmother
taught you a little song about lambs, frisking
in a pen, and you danced a silly little dance
with your grandmother, while the two of you
sang. So you sing it
for him, here in the dim, institutional
light of the hallway, light which even you
find insupportable, because even those who just
work here, and can leave when their
shift ends, deserve light to
see by, and because it reminds you
of the light in the hallway
outside the room
where, when your grandmother
dies, you were three thousand miles

away. So that you're singing the little song
and remembering the silly little dance
to console yourself, and to pay your grandmother
tribute, and to try to charm Polanski,

which you do; you sing, and Mr. Polanski,
he who had set himself against the doorjamb

to resist you, he who had made of himself
a fist, Mr. Polanski,
> *contentious, often*
> *combative and always*
> *and finally*
> *inconsolable*
hears that you know
the song. And he steps out
from the battlement
of the doorway, and begins to
shuffle

and sing along.   *(pp. 35–36)*

In capturing this moment through poetry, Krysl made substantial that which was seemingly insubstantial or invisible. As Gadamer (1988) said, we are "witness to our own being" (p. 115).

As part of the postmodern constructivist mode to ground human science as method, as science, and even as a form of feminist scholarship, poetry, story, and narrative have all been used as ways to decenter the unreflexive self so as to create a position for experiencing the self as an engaged knower/constructor. Such decentering reveals a way to (re)write the self as well as to unite people's (inter)subjective experiences with individual interpretations. This agenda for the interpretation of lived experience allows the paradigm to be inverted; human experience thus is pursued from the inside out, from the unconcealed poetic-aesthetical language model rather than from the outside, closed, concealment model of traditional scientific language systems. As a result, not only are new clearings opened, but there is evidence of poeticizing as eliciting truth.

One contemporary approach to considering poetry as a form of Truth is to take as its subject matter the lived experience of the researcher rather than the external data per se. Considering the life world of the researcher involves an epistemic shift within and across disciplines that joins a growing genre of research framed as Interpretive Biography (Denzin, 1991), Ethnographic Fiction

(Richardson, 1992), Radical Hermeneutics (Caputo, 1987), Radical Empiricism (Jackson, 1989), Transcendental Phenomenology (Levin, 1983; Watson, 1985), Interpretive Hermeneutics (Gadamer, 1988; Habermas, 1983), Story as Method (Boykin & Schoenhofer, 1991; Coles, 1989), and so on. This interpretative turn is one result of our disenchantment with the "modern structuralist era" of science and scientism, which we are now leaving behind as we enter into the postmodern era. More important than any postmodernism, however, is the search for ontological and epistemological authenticity as a form of Truth, with respect to the phenomena of interest *and* its human expression (Guba & Lincoln, 1989).

Specifically at issue is ontological authenticity in relation to the human-to-human transpersonal and contextual field in which nursing research (as praxis) finds itself with respect to the conditions and experiences of being human. For example, although nursing research may attempt to capture the descriptive meaning of the subjective lived experiences of patients as part of a qualitative research paradigm (e.g., phenomenology, ethnoscience, hermeneutics), the empirical context of traditional science still looms large, keeping the focus external (even though subjective) and directed toward the "other" out there. Little attention is given to the transaction per se, as if it were secondary to the phenomena of interest, its only purpose to inform the researcher about the "other's" experience. Within a postmodern frame and when considering poeticizing as Truth, there is another way to think about this situation. First, we can admit that it is never possible to *know* another person's experience; even though we may intuit it and vicariously identify with it, it remains uniquely *other*. Second, we can find it possible to *grasp* the other's experience by becoming better acquainted with how we encounter it as researcher, as clinician, and so on.

By inverting the paradigm and understanding human experiences from the inside out, we come full circle—from modern, detached, sterile language to postmodern connections, interpretations, and aesthetics. We see the beginning of a new dynamic of understanding human experience. Nursing's subject matter becomes, for nursing, authentically and even poetically expressed.

This ontological and epistemological turn helps nurse researchers keep conceptually consistent with the recent postmodern shifts that researchers are making across many disciplines. Further, it allows nursing to be ontologically and epistemologically authentic with respect to its history and tradition as well as to its most contemporary human caring, healing, and health care experiences. In doing so, it sets up another consideration for the treatment of researchers' data on the subjective human experience. This is perhaps where the question of poeticizing and Truth comes most dramatically into play.

THE QUESTION OF POETICIZING AND TRUTH

Facts can be considered as scientific knowledge only after passage through an authentication process. If perhaps the leaders thought more in terms of lasting values and ART, then science and knowledge would follow. (Polanyi, 1962)

Once we seek ontological and epistemological authenticity with the human experience in question, then we must consider authentic languaging to capture that experience. For Heidegger, the result is poeticizing—indeed, if the researcher engaged in and was reflective of the depth of the human experience, it cannot be other than poetic. Levin (1983) noted that, in phenomenological discourse, "the deepest transcendental truth of an existentially authentic languaging of experience will be articulated naturally with the sensuous resonance, the emotional spaciousness, and the elemental openness of the poetic word." Heidegger also urged that as we actually undergo an experience with language, we create an authenticity whereby the experiences speak for themselves. In the process, we should let ourselves be transformed by our participation. If the researcher is true to the moving human experience, he or she almost naturally poeticizes.

With respect to the Truth of poeticizing human experiences, once we acknowledge the authenticity and transcendental nature of both the experience and the nature of its expression, it is necessary to acknowledge that the way in which the experience is expressed is at least as important as the content, the facts, and the pure description of the experience (Watson, 1985, pp. 91–93). In other words, how could cold, unfeeling, detached, dogmatic words and tone possibly reveal the Truth or depth of meaning of a human phenomenon associated with transpersonal caring or convey the sorrow, great beauty, passion, and joy that are present. We cannot convey the complexity of the need for compassion or of the cultivation of feeling and sensibility in words that are bereft of warmth, kindness, and empathy. Within this paradigm is poetic ambiguity; we must learn to accept that. But such languaging itself invokes the very act of bringing the Truth of an experience into being. As a form of truth-telling, poeticizing is authentic to the ambiguity of human life itself. To quote Levin (1983):

> *If there be any truth, then [in the method] it must be that the transcendental is not just a method for understanding the facticity of experience; but that it is also a way of enjoying, or appreciating the intrinsically creative and open nature of experiences, because appreciation of this nature is a necessary condition for true and authentic existential knowledge.*

Authentic languaging is intimately involved in the potential for growth implied in our lived and felt transaction within the research experience as well as in our reflection-upon-experience. This difference is not so much a question of different contexts of meaning as one of ways of relating to the experiential process. We may seek to construct this newfound subjectivist–intersubjectivist truth via expanding our horizons of meaning and insights, but we discover this truth by fully actualizing our past and our newfound future, which is embedded in humanity, human meanings, language, and experience. Finally, we enter into Truth as a form of poetic justice when we reconnect with who and what we have become as humans—cocreators of ourselves and our discipline, as we are cocreators of science and art. At last, we know that we grasp a new Truth, one in which we can dwell.

REFERENCES

Ammons, A. R. (1983). Poetics (1971). In *Norton anthology of poetry* (p. 664). New York: Norton.

Bachelard, G. (1964). *The poetics of space.* (Maria Jolas, Trans.) Boston: Beacon Press.

Boykin, A., & Schoenhofer, S. D. (1991). Story as link between nursing practice, ontology, epistemology. *Image: The Journal of Nursing Scholarship, 23*(4), 245-248.

Caputo, J. D. (1987). *Radical hermeneutics.* Bloomington: Indiana University Press.

Coles, R. (1989). *The call of stories.* Boston: Houghton Mifflin.

Denzin, N. K. (1991). Representing lived experiences in ethnographic texts. In N. K. Denzin (Ed.), *Studies in symbolic interaction, Vol. 12.* Greenwich, CT: JAI.

Gadamer, H. G. (1991). *Truth and method* (2nd rev. ed.). New York: Crossroad Publishing.

Gadamer, H. G. (1988). *The relevance of the beautiful and other essays* (Robert Bernasconi, Ed.). New York: Cambridge University Press.

Gadow, S. (1990). *Beyond dualism: The dialectic of caring and knowing.* Paper presented at the International Caring Conference, Houston, TX.

Guba, E., & Lincoln, Y. (1989). *Fourth generation evaluation.* Newbury Park, CA: Sage.

Habermas, J. (1983). *Knowledge and human interests* (J. J. Shapiro, Trans.). Boston: Beacon Press.

Heidegger, M. (1971). *Poetry, language, thought* (A. Hofstadter, Trans.). New York: Harper & Row.

Heidegger, M. (1977). *Basic writings* (J. G. Gray & J. Stambaugh, Eds.). New York: Harper & Row.

Hofstadter, A. (1975). Translations and introduction to M. Heidegger, *Poetry, language, thought.* New York: Harper & Row.

Jackson, M. (1989). *Paths toward a clearing: Radical Empiricism and Ethnographic Inquiry.* Bloomington: Indiana University Press.

Keats, J. (1983). Ode on a Grecian urn (1819). In *Norton anthology of poetry* (p. 664). New York: Norton.

Koestler, A. (1968). *Ghost in the machine.* New York: Macmillan.

Krysl, M. (1989). Sunshine Acre Living Center. In *Midwife and other poems on caring.* New York: National League for Nursing.

Levin, D. (1983). The poetic function in phenomenological discourse. In W. L. McBride & C. O. Schrag (Eds.), *Phenomenology in a pluralistic context* (p. 221). Albany, NY: SUNY Press.

Marx, L. (1964). *Machine in the garden: Technology and the pastoral ideal in America.* New York: Oxford University Press.

Merleau Ponty, M. (1962). *Phenomenology of perception.* London: Routledge & Kegan Paul.

Miller, M. (1989). *Between psychology and psychotherapy. A poetics of experience.* New York and London: Routledge.

Parker, P. (1987). Community, conflict, and ways of knowing. *The Magazine of Higher Education, 19*; 20-25.

Polanyi, M. (1962). *Personal knowledge.* New York: Harper & Row.

Richardson, L. (1992). The consequences of poetic representation: Writing the other, rewriting the self. In C. Ellis & M. Flaherty (Eds.), *Investigating subjectivity: Research on lived experience* (pp. 125-141). Newbury Park, CA: Sage.

Watson, J. (1985). *Nursing: Human science and human care.* New York: National League for Nursing.

Watson, J. (1986). Arts and humanities in nursing. Inauguration address upon the inauguration of Dr. Sheila Ryan as Dean of Nursing, Rochester University School of Nursing. Rochester, NY.

Watson, J. (1987). Human caring and aging. Paper presented at the Distinguished Lecturer Series in recognition of Georgeva Owens Ferguson. Catholic University of America.

Watson, J. (1987b). Nursing on the caring edge: Metaphorical vignettes. *ANS, 10*(1), 10-18.

Watson, J. (1988). New dimensions of human caring theory. *NSQ, 1*(4), 175-181.

Williams, W. C. (1983). Red wheel barrow (1923). In *Norton anthology of poetry* (p. 945). New York: Norton.

2

Developing a Method for Aesthetic Knowing in Nursing

Peggy L. Chinn

art   craft   artisan   craftsman   craftswoman
crafty old woman   craft show   craft fair   art fair
art gallery   art studio   craft shop   artist   fine arts
healer   nurse   healing arts   nursing arts   witchcraft
witch   midwife   witchcraft craze

The idea of art, like so many other ideas, has long been assumed (on one level) to be neutral and gender-free. After all, "artist" does not carry a gender meaning. However, as I hope is clear from the

The contributions to this work by others were substantial, and I gratefully acknowledge the participation of nurses, students, patients, and colleagues. I especially acknowledge the substantive collaboration of nurse artists Charlene Eldridge, Kathy Maeve, Gerry Cancienne, Judy Bersch, and Janet Kemp all from Denver, and Judy Lumby (Sydney, Australia).

19

opening litany, implicit assumptions of gender saturate not only this concept, but concepts that have long been associated with the idea of art. (Did you notice implications of worth and value in the litany? Did you find value—or diminished value—associated with gender?)

As Ehrenreich and English (1978) explained, the history of healing is grounded in women's experiences and knowledge. For over 300 years, women were persecuted, prosecuted, and killed in Europe, in part because they held the power to heal. They were called "witches" and charged with "witchcraft." Equally disturbing was the attempt to systematically erase women's knowledge of the healing arts from human memory itself. Subsequent to this 300-year atrocity, a similar attempt was made to remove its memory via a perception of history, promoted by men, that failed to account for women's experience. It is no accident that, during this period, the fundamental tenets of what we now know as science were also being formed and set into traditions. We often fail today to notice our ignorance of women's tradition of healing. We assume that the science of cure is the ultimate human achievement. We also assume that science and art are distinctly different, even contradictory, because we have lost the memory of when they were and could have been one.

In this chapter, I submit that the powerful move toward art in nursing has its roots in a deep remembering of the women who once practiced the fine art of healing. Art is not something that stands in opposition to science; it is part of science—indeed, it is part of all human experience. Art expresses what words usually fail to express. Art brings wholeness to human consciousness. Art is powerful, profound, moving, and deeply political. Art is both feared and revered because it moves consciousness into realms not imagined and realities not predicted. Art is also feared, and sometimes revered, because it is associated, in the depths of human consciousness, with women, with the ability to create, to generate, to bring forth life. Analogous to the act of birthing, art brings forth, out of the inner spirit, the essence of human imagination, that which has not existed before. Art expresses the powerful intentions of the human spirit to move—to create revolution, to break free of the constraints of political and social boundaries, to bring into awareness something that is possible but is not yet. Art is the mirror, the creator, and the record of each human culture.

As nurses turn to art as a medium for developing nursing knowledge in a new century, we turn to birthing the potential of women's healing knowledge. Art as medium, as act, as process, and as product becomes a carrier for wisdom rooted in the ages, for memory of lost skill, for energy as yet untapped. Art becomes the expression of yearned-for wholeness, not only in the sense of encompassing all of human health experience, but in restoring within those who are nurses the wholeness that comes with linkage to ancient healing traditions that are rooted in women's ways of knowing.

For a century (only a third of the time span of the European witchcraft craze), nurses have worked with courage and persistence in roles and relationships characterized as oppressive; sometimes called handmaidens, they were more like servants than powerful healers. Throughout the twentieth century, strong voices have spoken and continue to speak out against the oppressive conditions and the power imbalances that constrict what nurses do and how they do it. Typically, the issue or problem is defined as lack of autonomy, or lack of professional status, or the need for recognition of the value of nurses' work. Ironically, nurses have turned to the methods and ideals of science to gain legitimacy, status, and rightful acceptance for nursing knowledge and nurses' work. However, in modern culture, art and science have been ripped apart, and this move led nursing further into denial of the ancient tradition arising from women's healing arts, a denial sustained by unyielding pressures from within the "scientific" community.

I submit that, although science, professional autonomy, and similar accomplishments have been and continue to be important and valuable, nursing's struggle goes on because nurses have not brought to consciousness the systematic erasure of women's healing wisdom; we nurses have not recognized the significance of the loss of memory of women's art of healing. Turning to art as a way of "seeing" the present meaning and experience of nursing, we also begin to remember that which has been lost and to truly comprehend the wisdom of our knowing and doing.

EVOLUTION OF A NEW CONSCIOUSNESS

During the first 50 years of the twentieth century, nurse training began to shift from a form of apprenticeship to university-based educational preparation. Academic nurses were required to develop collective knowledge and skills in the traditional scientific method. They came to perceive this method as inherently valuable and important in reaching goals related to nursing practice, as well as personal, political, and academic goals. By the early 1950s, the notion of a nursing science had emerged, and nurses began to apply traditional, empiric methods from a wide range of disciplines to the study of problems in nursing. Out of this diversity emerged collective recognition of the value of differing points of view. At the same time, nurse scholars recognized the limits of any single existing methods, particularly the traditional methods of science (Chinn & Jacobs, 1987; Meleis, 1985).

In 1981, the possibility of challenging existing conceptions of science gained widespread attention in nursing with the publication of "Nursing Theory and the Ghost of the Received View," an article by Webster, Jacox, and Baldwin. During the early and mid-1980s, calls for a shift to an alternate view to overcome the limits of traditional science methods predominated in nursing literature (Allen, 1985; Benner, 1985; Chinn, 1985; Tinkle & Beaton, 1983). This shift paralleled trends in other disciplines. In particular, there were striking commonalities between the insights of nurse scholars and feminist scholars. Nurse scholars challenged the medical model and its pervasive and limiting (and sometimes erroneous) influence over the methods of study related to health and illness (Allan & Hall, 1988; Ashley, 1980; MacPherson, 1983). Feminist scholars challenged the androcentric bias that yields partial (and sometimes erroneous) accounts of human existence (Ecker, 1986; Greene & Kahn, 1985; Harding, 1986, 1987; Keller, 1985; Newton & Rosenfelt, 1985; Reinharz & Davidman, 1988; Weiler, 1988; Wheeler & Chinn, 1989). Like feminist scholars, feminist nurse scholars drew connections between seemingly diverse social and political concepts and "scientific" concepts, revealing foundational meanings that underlie choices in method and substance (that which is studied) (Chinn, 1989; Dzurec, 1989; Meleis,

1987; Moccia, 1988). Methods of scholarship that reflect alternate values and world-views began to be described and applied (Benner & Wrubel, 1980; Connors, 1988).

From nursing's well-established philosophic tradition comes an urgency for nursing to shift and expand its focus of scholarly inquiry. Specifically, nursing literature reflects claims of (1) the essential unity of mind and body, (2) a societal role that addresses human experiences of health and illness, (3) the uniqueness of each individual's development over time, and (4) the integral nature of the social and political context to nursing practice and human experience. Let us examine each of these claims.

Nursing literature has sustained a persistent view that subscribes to the *essential unity of the mind and body,* a view that can be attributed to the practice of nursing as an art (Chinn & Kramer, 1987; Nightingale, 1969) and that gives rise to dissatisfaction with traditional empirical methods (Leonard, 1989). In fact, a view of unity is often in direct conflict with the most "rigorous" standards of scientific excellence.

The science of nursing addresses *human experiences of health and illness* (Benner & Wrubel, 1989). Thus, methods used in nursing should include those that address ontology (being) as a foundation for addressing epistemology (knowing). As a human science and as a social role, nursing's concerns include human subjectivity. Understanding and interpretation of experience take precedence over explanations used for the study of material phenomena (Dzurec, 1989; Munhall, 1989; Sarter, 1987).

Philosophically, nursing views human beings and *every human experience as unique and developing over time.* This view conflicts directly with methods of traditional scientific inquiry, structured for discovery of lawlike generalizable "truths" that hold from one individual or situation to another. Given nursing's perspective, methods that emphasize truth as mutable and that value the richness of the particular and unique are better suited to nursing's interests (Sandelowski, 1986).

Nurses and nursing exist within a *changing social and political context that is integral to human experience* and that calls for reflection and challenge. This context is one of diverse and complex perspectives, interests, and needs existing in contradiction, confrontation, and unequal social/political relations (Stevens, 1989; Thompson, 1987). Further, nursing traditionally views human experience as characterized by development and change; nursing's goal is commonly described as helping people to develop to their fullest potential within a given context—a process of constant transformation (Moccia, 1985). To date, traditional methods of science have been inadequate to address phenomena that are "in flux" and in context. Where traditional methods include change and contextual factors, these factors are treated as separate or isolated entities apart from the primary entity of study, rather than as integral to the existence of the whole.

Carper's (1975, 1978) work on nursing's patterns of knowing represented a breakthrough that provided a way to envision possibilities for developing nursing knowledge beyond the limits of traditional science. Besides empirics, Carper identified personal knowing, ethics, and aesthetics as essential patterns in the whole of nursing knowledge. Building on her conceptualization, Chinn and Kramer (1994) outlined methods for developing each pattern of knowing in nursing, and for expressing or communicating that which is known. As forms of knowing, personal knowing and aesthetics can only be represented in symbolic forms such as actions, sounds, or pictures, or in metaphoric language such as poetry or story. Each pattern of knowing, and its methods, is distinguishable, and each is essential to form a whole of knowing. The art of nursing, or aesthetics, is particularly important as an integrative pattern. Art in its finest forms requires and builds on all other patterns of knowing, possibly extending beyond what has been described and named as "knowing."

AESTHETICS: THE ART OF NURSING

The art of nursing is the art/act of the experience-in-the-moment. It is the direct apprehension of a situation, the intuitive and embodied knowing that arises from the practice/praxis of nursing (Chinn, 1989). Art arises from the immediate embodied grasp of the situation, the tools or instruments with which the artist works, and the intuitive knowing of what is to be created in the act.

The original art/act arises from a non-discursive, aesthetic knowing that is unique to the moment. Like other art forms, some aspects of the original art/act can be represented symbolically through stories, photographs, drawing, or poetry. Criticism also has its place here; it is the process by which the aesthetic pattern of knowing becomes visible and is shown to be plausible. Criticism is analogous to the original art/act in that it draws on creative and intuitive possibilities. Yet criticism functions in a reflective realm that looks into the art itself, transcends the moment of the art/act, and provides for a communal, or shared, appreciation of the completed work. Wheeler and Chinn's (1989) description of the connection between criticism as used in the context of group interactions and criticism as used in the arts is particularly apt:

> [D]eveloping your art to its finest level depends upon your own and others' criticisms. This type of criticism identifies the meanings of your work and reveals what creative possibilities need to be further developed.
>
> The art critic brings to the art insights and interpretations that help others to appreciate more fully what the artist has done, and what the art means for the culture as a whole. The critic does not proclaim the "correct" view of the art, but does provide a well-informed, knowledgeable interpretation of the art that helps others understand the art better, even if they don't agree with the views of the critic. (p. 37)

The idea of criticism that is central for an aesthetic method in nursing is the close connection to practice—the art/act of nursing—and to what can be created in practice in the future. Criticism is deliberately grounded in nursing praxis, which is "thoughtful reflection and action that occurs in synchrony, in the direction of transforming the world" (Wheeler & Chinn, 1989, p. 1).

Benner (1984), Benner and Tanner (1987), and Benner and Wrubel (1989) have provided exemplary work related to the method and the substance of aesthetic knowing. In her first book, *From Novice to Expert: Excellence and Power in Clinical Nursing*

Practice (1984), Benner warned that "once we consider caring as artful (although I [Benner] agree that it is), we risk ignoring caring as a subject of scholarly inquiry . . . . Caring is embedded in personal and cultural meanings and commitments. Therefore, the strategies for studying it must take into account meaning and commitments" (p. 171).

In my view, it is proper to consider nursing as an art and as a science, and as a subject of scholarly inquiry (as Benner has done). Benner's work provides a grounding for the phenomenologic methods that contribute to a method for aesthetics. The method I have developed incorporates both phenomenologic methods and methods of criticism. This ensemble invokes community, where the social and political meanings of nursing praxis (theory and practice) have the potential to be integrated into a fullness of knowing.

AESTHETIC DESIGN AND METHODS: HERMENEUTICS AND CRITICISM

Aesthetic methodology draws on two areas of inquiry: (1) critical hermeneutics as applied in the human sciences and (2) art criticism derived from the humanities. Each area of inquiry is grounded in a world-view of human experience as unique, truth as mutable, and meaning as primary. In addition, both of these seemingly diverse areas view their method as a means for inspiring change, refinement, perspective, development, movement, and social relevance (Eagleton, 1984; Polkinghorne, 1983; Reinharz, 1983). Hermeneutics (defined as the science of interpretation in philosophy) and criticism (defined as the science of resymbolizing in the arts) converge to form a possible new method that can be developed to create new understandings of the art of nursing.

Phenomenologic hermeneutics, specifically that derived for nursing by Benner and Wrubel (1989) from Heidegger (1982), is based on perspectives that shift the focus away from mental representational processes to the "immediate grasp of a situation in terms of its meaning for the self" (Benner & Wrubel, 1989, p. 42). The immediate grasp of a situation is made possible by:

- Embodied intelligence that allows the person to move through time and space, experiencing situations in terms of meaning in direct, nonreflective ways.
- Background meaning that is given to each person, from birth, by the culture; although it is personal and individual, it is shared by and taken up from the culture, subculture, and family.
- Concern, which is involvement in and commitment to a situation because of what matters to the person.
- The situation, which changes over time and directly involves the person; the person both constitutes and is constituted by the situation (Benner & Wrubel, 1989, pp. 42–50).

This approach of using critical hermeneutics in the method for aesthetics is drawn from the work of Habermas (1973, 1979) and Freire (1970). In Freire's work, pictures and photographs are used as codifications to represent a situation, showing some constituent elements in interaction. These "coded situations" are full of meanings that are assigned by instincts, learning, culture, and personal needs.

Codifications (tangible items such as verbal or written vignettes, magazine ads, drawings, or photographs) represent situations that are familiar to individuals in a culture and must be neither too explicit nor too enigmatic. Codifications make it possible to examine other related themes.

"Decoding" is a critical analysis of the coded situation. In decoding, the specifics of a situation are externalized through discussion with others. Emerging themes bring forth interpretations and make explicit our real consciousness of the world (in this case, consciousness of the art of nursing). Through decoding discussions, views of the art of nursing change and perceptions expand. As in all hermeneutic methods, decodimg moves from the abstract to the concrete, from the parts to the whole and back to the parts (the hermeneutic circle). Codifications in the form of photographs or verbal vignettes provide a way to look at situations that participants represent as the art of nursing. The discussion/decoding process begins with a description of the situation and moves toward identifying themes and reexamining meaning. Photographs or vignettes also provide opportunities to reflect on specific situations while separated from the emotional investment of "being there" and distanced from the descriptors applied to the experienced embodiment in the situation.

For the decoding process, method draws on art (including literary) criticism, which is closely akin to the perspectives and the interpretive methods of hermeneutics. A perspective thus opens up that moves beyond the performance, the art, or the act-in-the-moment. This is a reflective art in itself, and it requires an interactive element between the artist/actor and the person giving the criticism (who can be the same person). The interpretive work of criticism requires the actor/critic to bring to conscious awareness those meanings of the culture, the situation, and the whole context, while incorporating technical, ethical, political, and personal perspectives. In effect, the perspectives of doing (being) and knowing are integrated.

The essential element that hermeneutics and art criticism share in common is the use of disciplined, deliberate study, the goal of which is to reveal essential meanings in the text, process, experience, or situation. The method is ordered yet creative, rigorous yet open, logical yet intuitive (Smith, 1989). It is "empathically critical, not in the sense of voicing disapproval of contemporary arrangements, but in the sense that it tries to distill the meaning of historical processes . . . in relation to existing tendencies towards a freer society." (Bleicher, 1980, p. 159).

The work of Jurgen Habermas (1973, 1979; see also Bleicher, 1980; Eagleton, 1984) has influenced the methods of hermeneutics and of criticism that are the basis of the aesthetic method. Unlike the work of Habermas, however, the method described here does not impose certain preconceived psychoanalytic or Marxian formats on the situation. By shifting the focus to the art of criticism as it is described in the humanities (Bleich, 1978; Eagleton, 1984; Showalter, 1985), we move more toward a method that is grounded in the immediacy and wholeness of human experience and creativity, or what is thought of as artistic (Schon, 1987). The perspective of the arts opens the mind and heart to possibility. It taps the deepest regions of the spirit, where the heart of the self can be felt, touched, nurtured, and inspired. At the same time, criticism that emerges from the arts approximates these canons, cited in Polkinghorne (1983), which ensure plausible interpretation:

1. The researcher accepts the autonomy of the phenomenon itself; it is not forced into preconceived interpretive schemes.
2. The researcher searches for an interpretation that makes the phenomenon maximally reasonable (sensible) or human.
3. The researcher seeks the greatest possible familiarity with the phenomenon, including its history, various components of meaning, traditions, and envisioned future.
4. The process of understanding moves back and forth between the part and the whole, the particular and the general (hermeneutic circle).
5. Through a fusion of the researcher's own situation and the phenomenon under study, the researcher shows the meaning of the phenomenon for the present situation. (pp. 236–237)

TRUTH AND GENERALIZABILITY; VALIDITY; AND PREDICTION

These three issues arise as concerns in most discussions of scholarly methods that depart from the traditions of science. They are central to the development of the aesthetic method, and they make explicit how aesthetics, as a pattern of knowing, is distinguished from traditional empirical methods.

Truth and Generalizability

Scholars of the traditional hermeneutic methods have written volumes about the nature of truth, the dilemma of objectivity and subjectivity in discerning truth, and how to discern the "correct" interpretation. In most accounts, the authors have maintained an either/or posture: either such-and-such is true (correct) or it is false (wrong). The views of Heidegger and Gadamer do not polarize true and false. For example, Heidegger maintained that truth occurs in engagement with the world—each person's engagements reveal a certain truth. Gadamer also assumed a relativistic view of truth, expressed through the individual's life-world language. Betti (cited in Polkinghorne, 1983, p. 229) criticized these views as representing a "standardless morass of relativity." However, the notions of "relativity" and of "truth" or "correctness" can only arise from a system of thinking that assumes an adversarial dichotomy: right vs. wrong or true vs. false. In the aesthetic method, a both/and view is assumed; truth and falseness, right and wrong can coexist or be perceived in a situation simultaneously. The act of bringing to awareness these both/and possibilities brings forth a fuller, richer understanding or interpretation (Heldke, 1988).

In the arts, truth is not merely the unique truth expressed by the artist. Rather, art begins with the assumption of a common, generalizable human experience. Unlike empirics, which seeks a generalizable outcome that can be established as truth, art begins with a deeply known truth of human experience (birth, death, fear, guilt, suffering, joy, excitement) and seeks expression of the infinite creative possibilities for experiencing or responding to the human experience. Assuming that creative possibilities could be "true" for any one individual, the artist seeks to represent, inspire, and bring forth that which is uniquely possible.

Validity

Closely related to the issue of truth is the problem of how to discern validity: Is something what it is claimed to be? As hermeneutic methods for the human sciences developed, this problem became the focus of a response to relativistic interpretations of "truth." Hermeneutic scholars returned to an objectification of interpretations and to a reconstruction of meanings based on imposed insights drawn from the "objective" perspective of the researcher and using criteria for judging the validity of an interpretation based on the narrowness of the class (of interpretive content), the number of members in it, and the frequency of the trait among those members (Polkinghorne, 1983). As aesthetics developed, however, these criteria to ascertain validity were seen to belong more appropriately to empirics, where the concern is to ascertain that something is what it is claimed to be. For aesthetic purposes, what something *is* can be more than one "thing" simultaneously. There is usually more than one meaning; each meaning amplifies or informs another.

Plausibility of meanings as conveyed through criticism rests with the emergence of consensus, where each interpretive view can be apprehended or appreciated by others. Each interpretation is plausible to the extent that it takes account of the fullness of meaning that is admissible, or relevant, to that perspective. No account is taken to be "better than" or "more accurate than" another; each account is taken to be what it is, given the perspective from which it comes. In the arts, any representation (e.g., painting, performance, poem) is what it is. It may not be a reality shared by the viewer or the critic. The community of artists and those who study the art engage in dialogue and criticism to explore the contexts, assumptions, and values from which the representation flows, and how the representation might change in different contexts. Consensus arises out of the "empathic move" that creates an appreciation for an interpretation or meaning that is not fully shared but is comprehended as plausible for the other. At the same time, the consensus process, and the criticisms that emerge from it, reflect and contain consciously chosen values, judgments, ethics, and preferences. This dimension of "bringing choice to light" makes possible the aesthetic parallel to prediction—the act of "futuring."

Prediction

Futuring is an alternative to the traditional notion of prediction in empirics. The purposes of science, including the human sciences, commonly take as givens the goals of description, explanation, and prediction. Hermeneutics in general, and Heideggerian hermeneutics in particular, moves away from scientific goals that tend to assume objectified and distanced means–end dichotomies. Rather, the hermeneutic aim is simply to reveal the meaning that *is* in the human life realm. The method of aesthetics developed here draws on a meaning that emerges from temporality (the grounding of human experience in time) to move toward a collective process of "futuring." Unlike prediction, which presumes the ability to pre-scribe or control what might happen next, criticism is concerned with bringing alternative possibilities to full awareness in order to nurture the ability to shape a preferred future as a conscious, eth-ical, human choice. Criticism, like interpretive hermeneutics, illu-minates the nature of experience in the world but moves more fully into exploring multiple perceptions and possibilities within that experience, thereby revealing new possibilities for the future.

AESTHETIC EXPERIENTIAL CRITICISM: A METHOD FOR AESTHETICS IN NURSING

The method of aesthetics that I am advocating is also influenced by the work of feminist sociologist Shulamit Reinharz (1983), whose "experiential analysis" method was developed for the study of social phenomena. Aesthetic experiential criticism, like Rein-harz's experiential analysis, places the experience of the research at the center; the perspective of the investigator and the evolving experiences of the research itself are integral as "data" and are therefore subjected to the same degree of analysis as the substan-tive "data" of the study. This integration of the experience of the investigation itself makes possible, to the fullest extent, the inte-gration of context and meaning.

An exploratory study, begun in January 1992, continues to de-velop the methods of aesthetic experiential criticism. Described below are the refinements of these methods as effected in three acute-care settings with volunteer nurse participants. Specific fea-tures of aesthetic experiential criticism as method are detailed in the remainder of this section.

1. *Articulating the art/act of nursing and integrating self-reflective processes into the descriptions.* Practicing nurses work with the academic investigator (AI) as a coparticipant in this experiential phase of the process. The process begins with becoming mutually acquainted: the AI is oriented to the nurses' practice world, and they are oriented to the academic world.

Together, they decide on the best way to begin, evaluate the talents they can bring to the study situation and plan how they will draw on their nursing practice and on the AI's academic skills to articulate the art/act of nursing. One necessary element for sharing the meanings derived from the culture of nursing and developing the shared experiences of the art/act of nursing is the AI's becoming immersed in the practice situation. Together, the group seeks the participation of other people in specific situational events that have been mutually chosen for study. An overriding purpose of participation is to allow for varying individual descriptions of perceptions—what happened—and the meaning of the experience from individual points of view. Written notes and audio tape recordings of verbal interactions are used to form ongoing documentation of the discussion. From these are extracted by transcription the verbal vignettes that are selected as codifications of the art/act of nursing. The group also selects situations that have been identified to photograph; some are spontaneous and others are staged. The nurses share written stories of experiences that they identify as representations of the art of nursing. The processes of representation continue until the group is satisfied that it has sufficient material with which to work. Critical and creative insights emerge cooperatively within the process of gathering the vignettes or photographs. Discussion then focuses on self-reflective meanings of the situation, and the group explores the many meanings that coexist, some shared and some not shared.

   2. *Developing personal journaling as a tool for self-reflection and criticism.* Each participant initiates a journal, following guidelines developed by Hagan (1989). The participants/nurses sometimes choose to keep a personal journal as well. The journals are considered the private possessions of their authors. A "code of ethics" for journaling, developed by the Faculty of Nursing of Deakin University in Australia, is used as a guide for sharing the content of the journals and using it in the analysis and the report. Journaling is primarily self-reflective, but journal entries are brought into the experiential process by reading excerpts to other participants as a way of placing before the group possible meanings, metaphors, and symbols that arise from reflection.

3. *Documenting criticism as both substantive process and method.* The development of criticism is an ongoing process throughout the experience, but here (unlike empirical data analysis) the critic does not necessarily seek to develop all thematic insights possible. Rather, the critic focuses on compelling insights that have value for developing the art in the future.

Individual criticism develops from reflections on narrative vignettes, photographs, or other material representations shared in discussion, or from direct observation of a nurse's practice. The reflections, often recorded during journaling, are presented for group discussion. Criticism focused on a specific art/act is judged to be adequate when it (1) expresses metaphoric meaning of the art/act that expands consciousness of the art/act, (2) provides insight concerning the quality of the technical aspects of creating the art, and (3) gives the artist a frame from which to inspire further creative potential.

When insights become compelling and are repeated over time, the criticism is formalized and documented for future reflection. During documentation, the criticism is refined to ensure its completeness and adequacy. Complete formal criticism includes:

- Explanation of the historical, cultural, and political contexts in which the art is placed.
- Interpretation of technical (empiric) skills made visible in the art/act.
- Revelation of the critic's personal insights and history, from which insights arise.
- Ethical meanings symbolized in the art/act.
- Metaphors that express deeper meanings embedded in the art/act.
- Specific directions that the critic envisions for future creative development of the art.

4. *Developing consensus with respect to criticism.* The consensus arises from the experiences of the actors, which are recognizable as plausible even when the criticism is not one's own. All

participants review the criticism that emerges from the work done together. They then amplify any dimensions of the criticism that require further insight in order to clarify the perceived plausibility. As new critical insights are encountered, the individual actor of the experience is asked to confirm the plausibility, from a personal perspective, of the critical representation of the experience.

Preliminary Criticism

This research in progress grew initially from a conviction that the ways of science were not fully adequate to develop the knowledge of nursing. Initially, I did not see a connection between my interest in developing a "method" for aesthetic knowledge in nursing and my feminist insights. One was my academic life; the other *was* my life. It did not take long, however, for me to begin to see the deep connections between the two. In my work with the nurses who practice the art of nursing, several important insights have clarified these connections.

The art of nursing is closely connected with our bodies. Our bodies constitute the "carrier" of our art—they tell the story, convey the message, and portray the experience. For women, this realization has tremendous implications. Our existence as women has been epitomized as our bodies, and women's bodies have been bought, sold, and used to buy and sell. They have been the object of art, but, more importantly, they have become the decorative element of the crowd—painted, shaped, and twisted daily to conform to certain appearances, and to "sexualize" or "genderize" us in ways that we associate with feminine attractiveness and beauty. In part because of the overwhelming cultural emphasis on women's bodies, when we enter situations as nurses we bring with us a certain body-consciousness, or body self-consciousness, that is reflected in how we use our bodies in our art. The nurse artists in this study—women and men—have become sensitized to the ways their feelings and attitudes toward their own bodies have robbed them of potential to develop their art to its fullest. In many of our discussions, we reflected on this effect and imagined what it might be like to be able to use our bodies, as we envision we can, in developing our art to its fullest.

The significance of body posturing and body moves gives form and shape to the artistic essence of nursing.

Touch, both physical and symbolic, has emerged as a central element in the expression of nursing's art/act. We have not yet reached full understanding of the ways in which artistic touch is distinguished from technical touch, but nurse artists, without doubt, are making such a distinction. Predominant in our present awareness is the characteristic of enfolding or encircling. Some physical moves invite; they open a circle to embrace a situation. Others hold the circle: the caregiver leans over the person being cared for and administers the care with an open body position and a direct frontal gaze. Some closing moves—for example, a gentle pat or stroke—communicate that a door remains open to the future. Other closing moves communicate that all doors are closed. When a nurse feels threatened, fearful, or repulsed by a situation, the nurse's body visibly stiffens and moves backward almost imperceptibly.

We have begun to have new insights concerning the source of creativity, of aesthetic knowing, for the art of nursing. In contrast to early descriptions that associated aesthetic knowing in nursing with the phenomenon of empathy, we now suggest that the art of nursing and what constitutes the focus for developing aesthetic knowing originate from a similar space within the artist. Empathy, which requires a focus on and a move into the experience of "the other," is seen by nurse artists as interfering with creative potential, sustaining a diagnostic or therapizing mode of being that is *not* found in our explorations of what they experience as their art. Nurse artists recognize that, at times, empathy as a tool is necessary and valuable; when bringing "diagnostic" skill to their practice, empathy is essential. But when they practice their art as art, this is not what they are doing. Rather, the encounters that call forth what they most clearly associate with the art of nursing are those in which an apprehension of the meaning of a moment occurs without cognitive awareness. An instantaneous grasp of the situation and a simultaneous knowing call forth something from deep within the nurse. When such an artistic moment occurs, it is distinct from any sense of empathic understanding. Nurse artists describe these occasions as feeling within themselves something that moves to create an act; a situation generates spontaneously a feeling of "rightness." These occasions are sometimes attributed to intuition, but, after reflection, their meaning seems to have been informed by experience, by literature, and by all other forms of knowing—empiric, ethical, and personal. Consistent with definitions of the meaning of other art forms, nursing as art is expressive of a deep understanding of common human experience; its expression arises from within the creative wellspring of the nurse.

Like other descriptions of women's ways of knowing and being in the world, aesthetic knowing that gives life to the art of nursing does not grow out of reasoned, systematic, linear, problem-solving modes of thinking or action. Rather, aesthetic knowing involves an embodied grasp of situations and intimate experience with the deepest and most significant life events that have been traditionally and cross-culturally associated with women's experience— birth, death, sorrow, joy, pain, life transitions. Like artists in other forms of improvisational art, nurse artists know that they can perform spontaneously and with finesse only because of their practiced skill in ways of being and doing that are called for in the moment. As we develop in-depth descriptions of the art of nursing, we imagine more deliberate development of that practiced skill: "rehearsal stages" and "studios" where we examine the effect of working on the performance of the art. Such facilities would create an environment for rehearsing body moves and responding to situations where a "coach" can reflect on the performance and give direction and encouragement for trying alternate moves until knowing is achieved with an ensemble of body, mind, and spirit.

CONCLUSION

We stand on the threshold of developing knowledge of the art of nursing, and aesthetic knowing in nursing. Breaking new ground is difficult because the ways we have learned to think, to practice, to be, stifle creativity and devalue ways of knowing closely associated with women. As nurses engaged in the process of developing experiential criticism have reflected time and again, moving to new awareness of nursing practice as an art opens remarkable possibilities for the future.

REFERENCES

Allan, J. D., & Hall, B. A. (1988). Challenging the focus on technology: A critique of the medical model in a changing health care system. *Advances in Nursing Science, 10*(3), 22-34.

Allen, D. (1985). Nursing research and social control: Alternative models of science that emphasize understanding and emancipation. *Image: The Journal of Nursing Scholarship, 17*(2), 58-64.

Ashley, J. A. (1980). Power in structured misogyny: Implications for the politics of care. *Advances in Nursing Science, 2*(3), 3-22.

Benner, P. (1984). *From novice to expert: Excellence and power in clinical nursing practice.* Menlo Park, CA: Addison-Wesley.

Benner, P. (1985). Quality of life: A phenomenological perspective on explanation, prediction and understanding in nursing science. *Advances in Nursing Science, 8*(1), 1-14.

Benner, P., & Tanner, C. (1987). Clinical judgment: How expert nurses use intuition. *American Journal of Nursing, 87*(1), 23-31.

Benner, P., & Wrubel, J. (1989). *The primacy of caring: Stress and coping in health and illness.* Menlo Park, CA: Addison-Wesley.

Bleich, D. (1978). *Subjective criticism.* Baltimore: The Johns Hopkins University Press.

Bleicher, J. (1980). *Contemporary hermeneutics: Hermeneutics as method, philosophy and critique.* Boston: Routledge & Kegan Paul.

Carper, B. (1975). *Fundamental patterns of knowing in nursing.* Doctoral dissertation, Teachers College, Columbia University, New York.

Carper, B. A. (1978). Fundamental patterns of knowing in nursing. *Advances in Nursing Science, 1*(1), 13-23.

Chinn, P. L. (1985). Debunking myths in nursing theory and research. *Image: The Journal of Nursing Scholarship, 17*(2), 45-49.

Chinn, P. L. (1989). Nursing patterns of knowing and feminist thought. *Nursing & Health Care, 10*(2), 71-75.

Chinn, P. L., & Kramer, M. K. (1994). *Theory and nursing: A systematic approach* (4th ed.). St. Louis: Mosby.

Connors, D. D. (1988). A continuum of researcher-participant relationships: An analysis and critique. *Advances in Nursing Science, 10*(4), 32-42.

Dzurec, L. C. (1989). The necessity for and evolution of multiple paradigms for nursing research: A poststructuralist perspective. *Advances in Nursing Science, 11*(4), 69–77.

Eagleton, T. (1984). *The function of criticism: From the spectator to poststructuralism.* London: Verso.

Ecker, G. (Ed.). (1986). *Feminist aesthetics.* (Harriet Anderson, Trans.). Boston: Beacon Press.

Ehrenreich, B., & English, D. (1978). *For her own good: 150 years of the experts' advice to women.* New York: Anchor Press/Doubleday.

Freire, P. (1970). *The pedagogy of the oppressed.* New York: Seabury Press.

Greene, G., & Kahn, C. (Eds.). (1985). *Making a difference: Feminist literary criticism.* New York: Methuen.

Habermas, J. (1973). *Theory and practice.* (J. Viertel, Trans.). Boston: Beacon Press.

Habermas, J. (1979). *Communication and the evolution of society.* (T. McCarthy, Trans.). Boston: Beacon Press.

Hagan, K. L. (1989). *Internal affairs.* Atlanta, GA: Escapadia Press.

Harding, S. (1986). *The science question in feminism.* Ithaca: Cornell University Press.

Harding, S. (Ed.). (1987). *Feminism and methodology: Social science issues.* Bloomington: Indiana University Press.

Heidegger, M. (1982). *The basic problems of phenomenology.* (A. Hofstader, Trans.). Bloomington: Indiana University Press.

Heldke, L. (1988). Recipes for theory making. *Hypatia: A Journal of Feminist Philosophy, 3*(2), 15–29.

Keller, E. F. (1985). *Reflections on gender and science.* New Haven, CT: Yale University Press.

Leonard, V. W. (1989). A Heideggerian phenomenologic perspective on the concept of person. *Advances in Nursing Science, 11*(4), 40–55.

MacPherson, K. I. (1983). Feminist methods: A new paradigm for nursing research. *Advances in Nursing Science, 5*(2), 17–25.

Meleis, A. I. (1985). *Theoretical nursing.* Philadelphia: Lippincott.

Meleis, A. I. (1987). Knowledge development: Visions and re-visions. *Scholarly Inquiry for Nursing Practice, 1*(1), 11–20.

Moccia, P. (1985). A further investigation of "Dialectical Thinking as a Means of Understanding Systems-in-Development: Relevance to Rogers' Principles." *Advances in Nursing Science, 7*(4), 33–38.

Moccia, P. (1988). A critique of compromise: Beyond the methods debate. *Advances in Nursing Science, 10*(4), 1–9.

Munhall, P. L. (1989). Philosophical ponderings on qualitative research methods in nursing. *Nursing Science Quarterly, 2*(1), 20-28.

Newton, J., & Rosenfelt, D. (Eds.). (1985). *Feminist criticism and social change: Sex, class and race in literature and culture.* New York: Methuen.

Nightingale, F. (1969). *Notes on nursing: What it is and what it is not.* Unabridged republication of first American edition (D. Appleton and Company, 1860), with new preface by M. B. Dolan and Foreword by V. M. Dunbar. New York: Dover Publications.

Polkinghorne, D. (1983). *Methodology for the human sciences: Systems of inquiry.* Albany, NY: SUNY Press.

Reinharz, S. (1983). Experiential analysis: A contribution to feminist research. In G. Bowles & R. D. Klein (Eds.), *Theory of women's studies* (pp. 162-191). Boston: Routledge & Kegan Paul.

Reinharz, S., & Davidman, L. (1988). *Social science methods, feminist voices: Readings and interpretations.* New York: Pergamon.

Sandelowski, M. (1986). The problem of rigor in qualitative research. *Advances in Nursing Science, 8*(3), 27-37.

Sarter, B. (1987). Evolutionary idealism: A philosophical foundation for holistic nursing theory. *Advances in Nursing Science, 9*(2), 1-9.

Schon, D. A. (1987). *Educating the reflective practitioner.* San Francisco: Jossey-Bass.

Showalter, E. (Ed.). (1985). *The new feminist criticism: Essays on women, literature, and theory.* New York: Pantheon.

Smith, M. C. (1989). Facts about phenomenology in nursing. *Nursing Science Quarterly, 2*(1), 13-16.

Stevens, P. E. (1989). A critical social reconceptualization of environment in nursing: Implications for methodology. *Advances in Nursing Science, 11*(4), 56-68.

Thompson, J. L. (1987). Critical scholarship: The critique of domination in nursing. *Advances in Nursing Science, 10*(1), 27-38.

Tinkle, M. B., & Beaton, J. L. (1983). Toward a new view of science: Implications for nursing research. *Advances in Nursing Science, 5*(2), 27-36.

Webster, G., Jacox, A., & Baldwin, B. (1981). Nursing theory and the ghost of the received view. In H. K. Grace & J. C. McCloskey (Eds.), *Current issues in nursing* (pp. 26-35). Boston: Blackwell Scientific Publications.

Weiler, K. (1988). *Women teaching for change: Gender, class & power.* South Hadley, MA: Bergin & Garvey.

Wheeler, C. E., & Chinn, P. L. (1991). *Peace and power: A handbook of feminist process* (3rd ed.). New York: National League for Nursing.

3

Narrative Inquiry in Nursing

Toni M. Vezeau

If the world were clear, art would not exist.

Albert Camus

*I also write because I think one must not only
share what one thinks, or the conclusions one has
reached, but one must also share to help others
reach their conclusions.*

Sonia Sanchez

*N*urses care for persons in variant facets of health and life transitions. Nurses attempt to be present to individuals who, in living, build coherence and find meaning in life experiences. The primary struggle for the discipline of nursing has been to develop a generalizable knowledge base for care without sacrificing regard for the individual.

That struggle has forced a questioning of nursing's philosophical foundations and methods of inquiry. The concern has been to

41

balance the ambiguous stance persons necessarily have toward the world as both objective and subjective. How can nursing develop knowledge about persons in health and transition that acknowledges that ambiguity?

This question has resulted in a paradigm debate. Researchers have felt compelled to choose sides or to develop formulas for blending the two postures (Guba, 1990; Knafl & Brietmayer, 1991; Lincoln & Guba, 1985; Morse, 1991; Nowakowski, 1990; Reinharz, 1990). Triangulation, however, does not offer a third view; components of both postures are added together in a collaborative fashion rather than maintaining an antagonistic relationship. Although there is a new fit to the methodological puzzle, only two camps are envisioned and nursing becomes locked in an insoluble riddle. Perhaps the key to continued discussion is to explore other paradigms, to enlarge our perspective on how one person can know another in health and transition (Guba, 1990). It is proposed here that narrative is a worthy place of exploration for nursing inquiry.

Narrative makes a mutual world where reader, a community of readers, and storyteller meet to share in multiple realities using simple, human, language in place of specialized jargon. As inquiry, narrative is intended to enlarge the vision of a particular experience. The storyteller contributes metaphors to extend understanding beyond literal connection and asserts the human meanings of events. Readers bring reflection and openness in allowing the "shock of recognition" (Preston, 1987; Younger, 1990). In this process, narrative demonstrates a profound weaving of human context and responses that provide a solid base for knowledge development in nursing.

In this chapter, I will make common ground for discussing narrative inquiry and nursing. Because I favor creative narrative (fiction), I want, first, to examine narrative in its generic sense as story. Because this proposal is novel to nursing, I feel it is necessary to broach another issue that is common to any method of inquiry: rigor.

Second, in this chapter, I explain why I propose the creation of fiction by nurses as aesthetic inquiry. Fiction is an appropriate conveyance for sharing the personal knowledge that nurses develop in caring for patients, which can lead to personal knowing on the part of the reader. Fiction can help us explore the inner space of nursing and create visions for our future.

WHAT IS MEANT BY "NARRATIVE"?

We all know what stories are. Since our earliest memories as children we have received others' realities and expressed our own through stories. Because narrative involves so much of our inner world, however, I want to clarify what I understand as important to narrative.*

Narrative is a representation of a personal reality, editorialized and discrete, as information is. Most narrative does not try to answer questions; its object is exploration. The usual outcome is not certainty about a phenomenon, but the discovery of salient questions about the phenomenon that were not envisioned prior to the narrative.

Narrative is greatly different from scientific inquiry. Traditional science considers the particular, the part, as the cleanest and simplest aspect to study. The part is distinctly measurable, but it is not thought to have value or meaning in itself; its value is contingent on what can be generalized from many like parts. Traditional science values the general, the typical, and the most common, specifically because the part cannot be trusted to yield reliable and valid truth.

Narrative reverses this figure–ground relationship by valuing the part for its own personal truth. In a sense, narrative tests the conventional wisdom, the theory, about a type of experience by presenting a particular situation. The storyteller and audience both determine consonance and dissonance between the unique and the experience of the universal.

It is important to understand that narratives are not solely particular instances. No knowledge can result from disconnected singular parts. Narratives can be deconstructed for particulars—

---

* For more extensive detail on this topic, see Vezeau, 1993a, which provides an examination of variant narrative forms used in nursing inquiry. Pertinent text has been excerpted for use in this chapter.

facts, style, scenery—and in this way be *other-directed.* Narratives can also be appreciated as a whole in which meanings and feelings are experienced and in this way be *inner-directed.* In most narratives, these two stances toward story are simultaneous with the particular instance emphasized in the figure–ground appreciation of the phenomenon.

Narrative is special in that there is a personal draw to story; it requires belief that the storyteller has knowledge and belief that there are those who might listen. At its core, narrative, whether spoken or written, involves a coming to know self-and-others and self-in-others by trusting in the possibility of connection among persons.

Storytellers undergo very personal epistemological processes as they pursue a story. They learn to live the lives of others, as they imagine them, and to become familiar with the exterior landscape of the context—the sights, sounds, and smells—as well as the interior landscape of the experience. They learn, through profound reflection and imaginary living, the personal truths that can be found in certain human conditions. An authentic story comes about when a storyteller's knowledge base demonstrates the breadth and depth of the human condition within a specific context.

Nursing's history of inquiry includes narrative approaches that develop personal knowledge rooted in clinical practice (Boykin & Schoenhofer, 1991). Through stories, patients inform us about their experiences of health and transition. Stories have also been essential in conveying nurses' knowledge of individuals to each other. Currently, nurse researchers are pursuing qualitative methods using interview techniques based in narrative knowing. Nursing is no stranger to narrative; it has always been a part of how we explore the shared world of our patients.

Characteristics of Narrative

Time.   Part of the work of narrative is to connect events in time so that we can make sense of them. Unlike most other forms of inquiry, however, narrative is not time-bound. All temporal frames, for both storytellers and listeners, are drawn on past, present, future, experienced, or imaginary. Ricouer (1985), a philosopher who has written extensively on the circle between time and personal narrative, stated:

> . . . *between the activity of narrating a story and the temporal character of human experience there exists a correlation that is not merely accidental but that presents a transcultural form of necessity. To put it another way, time becomes human to the extent that it is articulated through a narrative mode, and narrative attains its full meaning when it becomes a condition of temporal existence.* (p. 52, author's emphasis)

Le Guin (1989) also described this essential aspect of fictional narrative:

> *So narrative is used to connect events in time. The connection, whether conceived as a closed pattern, beginning-middle-end, or an open one, past-present-future, whether seen as lineal or spiral or recursive, involves a movement "through" time for which spatial metaphor is adequate. Narrative makes a journey. It goes from A to Z. . . . It asserts, affirms, participates in directional time, time experienced, time as meaningful. (pp. 38–39)*

The ability to structure experience into a beginning-middle-end narrative is basic. Because this relationship between time and narrative is also central to my discussion of rigor in narrative inquiry, I will revisit it in more detail later.

Active Inquiry.   Narrative is active inquiry. If there are other outcomes—entertainment, catharsis, fear—these are secondary to facing an initial question or problem. Storytellers develop a story to discover what is on the other side. They want to live in that place a bit longer until they know more—not all, but more. The same is true of those receiving the story. The process of living in the story, of questioning, is the primary goal of telling a story. Dillard (1989) observed:

A writer looking for subjects inquires not after what he loves best, but after what he alone loves at all. . . . Why do you never find anything written about the idiosyncratic thought you advert to, about your fascination with something no one else understands? Because it is up to you. . . . It is hard to explain because you have never read it on any page; there you begin. (pp. 67–68)

Healing Properties.   One of the most satisfying and least spoken about aspects of any kind of narrative is the capacity of humans to tell stories to heal themselves and others. By helping us make sense of our world, narrative allows us to live in it as participants and not combatants.

This need for narrative unity is beginning to be recognized in medical literature as a basic requirement for physical and mental health. Long (1986) made a strong point that health states must not be perceived as having only chronicity without narrative unity—without sense-making:

. . . misfortune can be nothing more than misfortune, unasked for and incomprehensible; each cries out: "Why me?", only to confront silence. But in a narratively unified life . . . such events are given significance. . . . (p. 80)

The work of health professionals may well be to promote narrative process in their patients (Livo & Rietz, 1986). This is consistent with the nursing theory of Watson (1985), which posits that human care occurs precisely when the meaning of previously incomprehensible events is developed jointly by the nurse and the patient.

Storytelling may set the stage for recovery, and, as nurses, we need to appreciate its value. . . . I believe nurses need to stay with the anxiety engendered in them by the stories they hear; they should not escape behind assessment guides or history-taking activities. Storytelling is more than entertainment or socializing. Storytelling helps patients find meaning in their experiences and gives them

*the opportunity to reconstruct their lives. Storytelling pro-
motes healing. (Bartol, 1989a, p. 565)*

Stories can create a harmony, a sense of congruence between the
self and the world, not only for the patient but for the caregiver as
well (Hillman, 1983). Perhaps story is so basic to humans because
it allows us to live in our world as engaged mortals, mediating
risks and untoward events with the hope and healing that are
within our power to evoke.

FICTIONAL NARRATIVE

Discrimination among different types of narrative is important if
we are to use them as inquiry that develops nursing knowledge.
The number of narrative styles is almost endless, but the primary
ones that nursing has used in inquiry are: journals, hermeneutics
entailing patient-as-text, interviews, paradigm cases, "telling your
own story," and fictional narrative. Each of these forms has important aspects to attend to and cannot be equated. A thorough discussion of this issue in narrative inquiry (see Vezeau, 1993a) is
beyond the scope of my topic here, but I will provide a brief clarification regarding fictional narrative.

Fictional narrative is a form of inquiry that examines a particular setting and an individual response to that setting in the swirl of
events of a specific time. In the telling of a story, the particular
and unique aspects of an experience are moved to the foreground
of attention against the backdrop of what the reader may have previously experienced or believes to be true. In the engagement of a
particular event, narrative can present the novel, the surprising,
and the morally complex, which can lead to enhanced understanding of that event. Through successful narrative, the grounding
(that which has been previously appreciated) is transformed for
the writer and reader.

Fictional narrative is inquiry that actively seeks new awareness, a new personal relationship to the issues raised in a story.
This type of inquiry is not rule-bound; it requires creative play
and deep reflection. Narrative exists not only to allow for the

experience of a reality previously unimagined or felt, but to prompt personal change.

Fictional narrative is the imaginative depiction of actual or imagined events, developed from personal sources and represented in first-, second-, and third-person accounts. Fiction operates in the conditional tense of action: "might have happened" or "could have happened." This type of story involves a way of stalking that requires a supple awareness of the form and intensity new knowledge might take.

> *In summer, I stalk. . . . I can stalk them in either of two ways. The first is not what you think of as true stalking, but it is the Via negativa, and as fruitful as actual pursuit. When I stalk this way I take my stand on a bridge and wait, emptied. I put myself in the way of the creature's passage, like spring Eskimos at a seal's breathing hole. Something might come; something might go. . . . Stalking the other way, I forge my own passage seeking the creature. I wander the banks; what I find, I follow, doggedly, like Eskimos haunting caribou herds. (Dillard, 1982a, pp. 187–188)*

Fictional narrative is not "true," in the scientific sense of provable. Within nonfiction text there is a "true" version. This is what is sought in journals and interviews—the teller's personal truth. There is an allegiance to historical facts which frame the story for the teller and the audience. The facts are addressed first by the teller and narratively "smoothed" to give the story a seamless appearance (Spence, 1982). Within a personal story are sureness, clarity, and homogeneity in terms of what an experience means (Robinson, 1990, p. 1173). Historically based stories aim, in part, to persuade the listener and to control the interpretation of the event. The meaning is prescribed as well as described because the teller is also the protagonist of the story.

Ricouer (1985), in his examination of narrative as inquiry, explained fictional narrative's claim to truth:

> *I am reserving the term "fiction" for those literary creations that do not have historical narrative's ambition to*

constitute a true narrative. . . . What historical narra-
tive and fictional narrative do have in common is that
they both stem from the same configuring operations
. . . . On the other hand, what opposes them to each other
does not have to do with the structuring activity invested
in their narrative structures as such, rather it has to do
with "truth-claim." (p. 3)

Fiction presents a parallel world; prior to the reading, there is
no shared environment of a lived historical event and there may be
no referent or actual occasion for comparison. Fiction stands
alone. It is not autobiography, and, often, not personal experience.
Even when fiction is sparked by a specific lived event, the story
bears little resemblance. There is no desire in fiction to say "This is
what really happened." The storyteller only says, "This is what
happens."

RIGOR IN FICTIONAL NARRATIVE

If narrative is to be understood as valuable in knowledge development, scholars must raise the issue of rigor. That is, if works of fiction are said to lead to knowledge, what are the standards to judge
the trustworthiness of story, and what is the nature of this knowledge? Because knowledge is used on behalf of others, it is morally
imperative that what is learned is faithful to human experience.

Scholars have misgivings about accepting narrative in the
sphere of knowledge development. There is a risk that, unless
these issues are understood, narrative will continue to be, at best,
trivialized and, at worst, suspect.

Rigor in the context of inquiry refers to the trustworthiness of
the results produced. If what is learned in the process and product
of narrative is valuable to nursing, there must be clarity as to the
conditions in which story can be taken to heart and attended to.

The standards of rigor for quantitative research methods are inappropriate. Narrative does not measure experiences.

The standards of rigor for qualitative research may be more
congruent with narrative because both qualitative research and

narrative involve interpretive knowing and reformulation (Sande-lowski, 1991). Still, the standards for qualitative research are insuf-ficient—it is not the intent of narrative to produce theory.

Ideas of truth value or credibility may be a part of trustworthi-ness in narrative. Sandelowski (1986) described credibility as a "faithful description of interpretation of a human experience" (p. 30). But credibility is too limited a focus: readers choose a story in order to have their reality challenged.

Applicability as a component of rigor refers to the ability to transfer results to a related context. As a standard for narrative, however, this is also inappropriate. The intent of narrative is to provide a unique interpretation of human experience. For this rea-son also, reliability or consistency is not germane to narrative.

Fiction has persisted as a worthy exploration and expression of human experience in all cultures and in all times. In tandem, the discussion of story as truth or lie persists as well. Once fiction is acknowledged as imagined, are stories inherently untrustworthy?

Harm and Evil in Narrative

Krysl (1991), a noted writer of prose and poetry, in speaking to this issue stated that a failure of our culture is that data are more important than story. Stories are like prayers that heal us. Stories are powerful, and Krysl states that stories hold power for good and evil. Once a story is told, it cannot be called back. Only a more powerful story can be told to overcome an evil story.

Scholars have questioned the power of stories to promote indi-vidual harm and societal evil. It is this viewpoint that has been the driving force behind science's struggle for certitude and unbiased knowledge claims. Because stories are essentially unfounded and imagined, perhaps scholars should remain skeptical of narrative as inquiry.

A French literary critic, Roland Barthes, says that narrative puts forth a moral perspective on the world toward the goals of power over and manipulation of the reader (see Carr, 1986). Therein lies narrative's power as well as its culpability in serious inquiry. White (1981) and Mink (1978), two noted literary critics, shared this view.

Apprehension over the seductiveness of aesthetic modes of inquiry is a common theme of caution whenever there is discussion of possible integration of art forms and praxis in medicine, law, and nursing. Gadow (1990) stated:

> *One of the most troublesome aspects of the aesthetic approach is that heightened aesthetic awareness and activity can take an appreciative attitude toward nearly anything. . . . The aesthetic approach can dwell quite easily on the most horrifying human experiences. By itself the aesthetic approach knows no moral code, submits to no external standards. (pp. 2-3)*

Because aesthetic form can "make beautiful" what is not beautiful in human experience, its outcome is not necessarily truthful. Gadow's primary concern with art is its lack of allegiance to morality. Gadow explained that aesthetic forms can be allied with nursing praxis only if art adheres to the moral code of caring. Otherwise, in his view, there is danger from the seduction of immoral representation. Skillful storytelling can be a seductive siren's call drawing us emotionally into places where we would not normally travel. Where beauty is the draw of a story, the purpose may be to distract us from immorality. In this way, story can be intentionally untruthful and used for power and manipulation.

These viewpoints are potentially damning of criticism of my proposal that narrative is a worthy mode of inquiry for nursing and is consistent with human caring. Are not the above concerns based on an overly narrow view of narrative and of what can be included as knowledge?

Knowledge and Narrative

Definitions of knowledge take many forms. Polkinghorne (1983), in his discussion of methodology for the human sciences, looked at the historically changing descriptions of knowledge. Knowledge has been defined generally within the scientific realm of human endeavors as "the true and certain understanding of reality" (p. 10). Positivism as a philosophy of science proposed skepticism about knowledge claims unless there was absolute—or, more recently, probabilistic—surety. In light of this proposal, our common realization of the world has been transformed into mere opinion. For the positivist, knowledge is secured from five-sense perception. Somehow, if we could keep our individuality, our humanness, sequestered from the exploration of our own territory, we could become knowledgeable about it. With the development of the human sciences, this rigid description of knowledge could not be sustained.

Postpositivist thinkers challenged this narrow view of knowledge by denying the notion that humans can stand outside language and culture to achieve an "absolute" viewpoint. Knowledge was conceived of as conditional and as dependent on preexisting interactive systems that are contextually and communally derived.

Dilthey (1900/1976), a primary postpositivist thinker, proposed an expansion of the notion of knowledge to include "Verstehen," commonly translated as understanding. Emphasis here is on the meaning of perception of the world. Verstehen involves a broadened awareness that is specific to its context. The assumptions of verstehen as a valuable and trustworthy form of human knowledge oppose positivist rigidity. Multiplicity of realities, constant change in realities, and the integrality of knower and known become predominant.

Verstehen is exceedingly resistant to purely logical analysis—it is not reducible to parts, of either an inductive or deductive nature. Verstehen is a process that involves the total engagement of a person with a specific context. There is a back and forth flow of encounter to create meaning. The knower first attends to an aspect of a situation, then leans back to apprehend the whole, then attends to a part, and so on. The process is not solely mental; it involves the whole person.

Simultaneous with the proposal of verstehen as a valuable form of knowledge came rules developed to establish validity. Because verstehen leads to a communication of what is understood, it is conceptualized and signified in language. There was a felt need for guidelines for valid linguistic representation of human experience, and hermeneutics was developed in response to that need. Polkinghorne (1983) explained hermeneutics as:

> . . . *the science of correct Understanding or interpretation. It provides an exposition of rules to guide successful Understanding so that the interpretive effort is more efficient and so that the validity of its results is safeguarded from the intrusion of arbitrariness and subjective misunderstanding. (p. 218)*

The focus of the inclusion of verstehen as knowledge was utilitarian. Ultimately, the purpose of verstehen was to effect change. Understanding would lead to explanations that would support social action.

Heidegger (1927) used hermeneutics for a different purpose. Whereas Dilthey saw hermeneutics as a tool to obtain objective understanding, Heidegger proposed understanding not as a tool but as the way humans naturally live.

Gadamer (1989), expanding on Heidegger's view of knowledge, maintained that verstehen is achieved by a kind of translation, as if from another language, in which text is not literally rendered word-for-word but is interpreted as a whole. This type of interpretation involves a "fusion of horizons" between the anticipations of the interpreter and the meanings in the text—always process, not product, and in revision.

I find it difficult to see nursing's relation to a utilitarian position on verstehen. The Heidegger/Gadamer conceptualization supports the open quality of verstehen that characterizes nursing—a good in itself because it provides a common place to live that allows for engagement among persons. Rules toward "correct" understanding are a posture in defense to positivism as the dominant paradigm of knowledge generation. Nursing in its most heartfelt clinical aspects relishes ambiguity. Not to be certain—to be, instead, open to new interpretations and new meanings—is to retain the mystery and uniqueness of an encounter, to trust in the slow unfolding of the world. Narrative can be a part of knowledge development for nursing when knowledge is expanded to include the human dimension of verstehen, which is not exact or static (Bartol, 1989b).

Aspects That Support Rigor

Communally Derived.   Fiction, although often communicated by an individual, is a communal product.

> *It brings us back to the traditional position of the storyteller in a community, which is not to be the wise person, the person who speaks from his own wisdom, but to create an atmosphere in which the wisdom inherent in the world becomes apparent. (Lopez, in Lueders, 1989, p. 23)*

Storytellers are not isolates; they are thinkers who communicate back to their world the concerns implicitly found. Stories can mirror a culture, but their power lies in the illumination of issues usually camouflaged; to some degree, stories must be both mirrors and lamps. The world responds to one story, and the storyteller is moved to tell another before attention and courage wane.

> *For masterpieces are not single and solitary births; they are the outcome of many years of thinking in common, of thinking by the body of the people, so that the experience of the mass is behind the single voice. (Woolf, 1929, p. 113)*

I contend that no story is thoroughly fictional. Can storytellers really make something out of nothing, and if they could, would anyone recognize it?

The materials of story are not something made out of nothing: the stuff of stories is life. The role that imagination plays is in the development of new combinations that compel one to stay and reflect. If all fiction were not based in the already-known territory of human experience, it would have no draw and no sustained encounter.

> *. . . fiction is like a spider's web, attached ever so lightly perhaps, but still attached to life at all four corners. Often*

the attachment is scarcely perceptible. . . . But when the web is pulled askew, hooked up at the edge, torn in the middle, one remembers that these webs are not spun in midair by incorporeal creatures, but are the work of suffering human beings, and are attached to grossly material things, like health and money and the houses we live in. (Woolf, 1929, p. 72)

Fictional narrative has persisted as a form of knowledge development because humans sense truth in its formulation of reality. The heart of fiction is not make-believe, but recognition.

Contrary to Ideology.   There are profound fears regarding the acceptance of story as valid human inquiry. We all have experienced intentional lies and inadvertent misunderstanding. In the absence of a lie-detector test, how can the truth of stories be reconciled with experiences of individual and social lies?

A story does not cling to a singular interpreted meaning, nor is it a well-debated argument that narrows to an inescapable conclusion. Story is not propaganda, not ideology. The core of propaganda and argument is persuasion; the listener is not engaged to think or to question. The world of lies is static, objective, and other.

Gadow, who locates danger in the acceptance of narrative knowing, uses nazism as an exemplar of evil wrought by story (personal communication, 1991). Gadow imagines a situation in which drunk nazis in a bar are convincing other patrons of the truth of their "story"—the necessity and worthiness of genocide and domination. This is not story but propaganda in disguise.

Nazism, as an exemplar of lies on a devastating scale, cannot admit to alternative endings or disagreement among themes. Those listeners who disagreed were killed. Lies are dogmatic, static, and inflexible; they are deaf dogs barking with a hell of a bite. Unlike lies, the meaning of a story is not predetermined and well outlined. It is not story if it is the only story.

Do most stories have a message? The power of story is its ability to evoke and, at times, to provoke, and some writers do use story not just as expression but as a tool. In this pragmatic tradition of art, the message may be primary and directed toward social action (Abrams, 1959; Higgins, 1976). A story can be a means to an end and is judged by its strength of message. Can story have a message and not be propaganda?

That all stories have some message is inarguable. Writers commit pen to paper to say something that they find important and meaningful. All writing is perspectival, and writers highlight the aspects of a situation that are most apparent and poignant to them. But the difference between propaganda and story is the difference between used-car sales and a conversation.

In story, the role for the reader is offered, not prescribed. A reader of a story can choose to freely interact with the story and defines a personal role and outcome. In propaganda, how the reader "should" think and behave is clear, and the reader finds it difficult to refuse the imposed role. One can put down a book, but a Jew was not free to leave Nazi Germany. Propaganda, if disbelieved, implies repercussions to the reader. A story offers a version of the world; propaganda mandates it through fear. Story does not intend to deceive; propaganda does. Story invites interaction with the reader; propaganda negates relation.

We learn to recognize the difference and to teach our children to do the same. Neither the sentence produced by the imagination nor the scientific method should be damned or disallowed as part of inquiry. Each needs to be considered with hope, openness, and alertness.

Co-creation of Meaning. Story emphasizes the role of the listener in determining the story. The storyteller may have started the interaction and put something new into the common space, but what the story means is not solely created by the author. Creation of meaning in narrative requires commonality and reciprocity among author, story, and audience.

Early communication theory attempted to understand this cocreation of meaning in narrative. Jakobson's (1960) essay "Linguistics and Poetry," a primary source of communication theory about narrative, outlined communication as a process in which an address is sent and then received. Of critical importance is the fact that there is no communication unless the address is picked up by an audience. Audience reception is based on a moment of contact and on mutual understanding of the code through which the address is communicated, the pattern of the message, and the clarity of the context. Success in communication requires competent functioning of the whole. For Jakobson, the address alone cannot supply meaning.

Meaning is established by the reader based on what is expected from the context of the story and what is found. There is a struggle between "the role offered . . . by the text and the real reader's own disposition" (Iser, 1978, p. 3). The writer speaks through the interactions of characters and through direct statements to the reader. The reader has to determine a cogent viewpoint that represents a convergence of perspectives: the personal sense of role dissonance, the characters' opinions, and the author's position.

Interpretation, the development of meaning of text, is then dependent on the reader. Because readers differ in social, cultural, and historical backgrounds, expectations, and skills, multiple interpretations of text result. Variability among readers causes a story to be enjoyed and understood by one person and not another.

Negative or bland reception of a story may not necessarily reflect a lack of skill in the writer; a breakdown in the communication event may have occurred elsewhere. If a story "works," the writer and the reader commonly locate the context and issues in the story, but the meaning of the story to the writer may still be radically different from its meaning to the reader.

Because of the intricate, complex nature of the land, it is not always possible for a storyteller to grasp what is contained in a story. The intent of the storyteller, then, must be to evoke, honestly, some single aspect of all that the land contains. . . . As long as the storyteller carefully describes the order before him, and uses his storytelling skill to heighten and emphasize certain relationships, it is even possible for the story to be more successful than the storyteller himself is able to imagine. (Lopez, 1988, pp. 69-70)

Trustworthiness of Narrative

Narrative answers a unique question: "What *can* it mean?" or "What *can* it be like?" rather than "What does it mean?" or "What is it like?" Narrative speaks only to possibilities.

> . . . *fictional stories do not represent reality because what they portray by definition never happened. But it is often thought that stories can be life-like precisely by virtue of form. That is, they are capable of representing the way certain events, if they had happened, might have unfolded. (Carr, 1986, p. 13)*

Narrative adds to the differential understanding of a situation within a specific context, but does not, and cannot, offer a definitive position for the reader. The assessment of rigor in narrative becomes "When is a story a story?", not the determination of "When is a story truthful?"

As they mature, all persons develop criteria by which they can distinguish among a story, an argument, and a lie. Although these criteria are not usually reflected on, they operate in all interactions and come to consciousness only when we are awakened by the threat of a lie. Criteria are unique to each individual—no two persons judge story and lie the same. What follows is my list of distinguishing criteria. The list is not all-inclusive; it reflects only what works for me. Such criteria are as fallible as any human inventions. They are not law but only suggestions to consider so that readers can be encouraged to uncover their own list.

Emotion.   In contrast to scientific accounting of phenomena, stories fully engage the reader. The reader's emotional capabilities are drawn on and used in the interaction with a story. A trustworthy story does not leave the reader dispassionate about the issues at hand. In the bringing of emotions to the task of understanding a story, the reader develops this aspect of being human to the betterment of all other faculties (Jaggar, 1989).

Plausibility.   A story must be believable in order to merit attention. Plausibility refers to the capacity of the reader to believe the story as well as the skill of the writer to produce a story that could have happened. In determining plausibility, a reader questions: Could it have happened to the characters and is it likely that they responded in that way? If there are surprises or dissonances that contradict my expectations, can I supply the missing pieces? If I am not given all details in the story—the color of a character's hair, or what a room smelled like—can I fill them in?

Feminist literary critics are discouraged by so much of the literary canon precisely on this notion of believability. Characters must be individuals. Too often, women are portrayed stereotypically and only in relation to male characters. Literature of the canon is rarely plausible in terms of yielding truth about women's lives. Female characters are shallow, unlikely, and without voices.

Plausibility is not a matter of whether *the reader* would behave in a particular fashion, but whether the world described in the book story is likely to, based on how it is presented by the author. Believability has to do much more with the reader's ability to recognize stereotyping, the rigidity of the reader's expectations, and the breadth of the reader's life experience. Plausibility is also influenced by the skill of the writer; it is dependent on an ability to suspend previous notions of the world to even consider a different one.

Details.   What helps to determine whether a piece warrants attention? The degree of details given (not their number but their intensity) to keep the reader from becoming lost in an unknown world. I cannot trust a story if I cannot recognize who these people are and the nature of the land. My ability to do this differs every day of the week and, as I get older, I trust more openly with fewer clues.

Awareness.   After reading a trustworthy story, I know more than before; I understand human experience more fully. I find in the story knowledge that changes my preconceptions or misconceptions about a world I thought I knew. A trustworthy story is not a mirror; it is a new world to live in, a changed world that I am returning to. To understand a human experience is to become a stranger to the world I just left.

Power to Elicit Personal Knowledge.   A true story, as opposed to a lie or propaganda, allows me to focus on my own life experience. I cannot do otherwise; it is why I attend (Gadow, 1990). I continue to read because I need to know how *I* will turn out as well as the story. In this way, the story invites me to include personal knowledge with the content of the text—in essence, to rewrite the story. Any story that prevents my voice and my personal life experience from entering is dangerous and suspect.

Lack of Certainty.   Honest fiction has a hesitant, porous quality. A true story is never the only story. If it is, what appears to be a story is something else—argument, lie, or propaganda. I do not sense coercion or persuasion. I can provide alternative endings and motivations.

Multiplicity of Interpretations.   A rigorous story should be able to spark debate among readers. Qualitative research, according to Lincoln and Guba (1985), generates knowledge based on scholarly consensus, but this could never be appropriate for narrative. There *should* be disagreement over the meaning of a story because the meaning is cocreated by the individual who reads it. If this does not happen in story, it is, again, ideology.

Yet a story is not a Rorschach inkblot. Authors provide context, details, and plot. There is at least some common understanding of events and characters. Without a shared map, readers could not interact. A true story combines obvious "facts" and, at times, obvious themes, but what they mean will always be individually interpreted and correct.

USE OF FICTION AS AESTHETIC INQUIRY WITHIN THE HUMAN SCIENCE OF NURSING

Nursing is attempting to define itself as science. Although it has been acknowledged that clinical nursing can also be an art, it is nursing as science that is credentialed and funded. Creative writing as inquiry is distinctly unscientific and, because scientific is presently equated with scholarly, it is generally considered unscholarly. Yet, all fiction is essentially experimentation with unique circumstances:

> *It [is] a heuristic device, a thought-experiment. Physicists often do thought-experiments. Einstein shoots a light ray through a moving elevator; Schrodinger puts a cat in a box. There is no elevator, no cat, no box. The experiment is performed, the question is asked, in the mind. Einstein's elevator, Schrodinger's cat, my [characters], are simply a way of thinking. They are questions, not answers; process, not*

*stasis. One of the essential functions of . . . fiction, I think,
is precisely this kind of question-asking: reversals of a habit-
ual way of thinking, metaphors for what our language has
no words for as yet, experiments in imagination. (Le Guin,
1989, p. 9)*

For all that has been written about aesthetic knowing (Benner
& Wrubel, 1989; Carper, 1978; Watson, 1985), little aesthetic inquiry has been encouraged or published. As stated in the chapter's
introduction, however, there is a need for nursing as a profession
that cares for individuals to develop a path of inquiry that uses aesthetic knowing of individual situations.

Nurses are beginning to develop poetry and prose to portray
lived experiences as they are lived. Fiction may be sparked by
events at the bedside, but nurse writers use imagination and their
wealth of engagement with others in health care settings to communicate context and meaning (Vezeau, 1993b). Tisdale (1986,
1988), an excellent example of a nurse writer, is well-known for
stories that combine historical actuality, imaginative extension
and embellishment, and technical information in a variety of nursing situations. There are few avenues to communicate fictional
writing for nurses, but I suspect that many nurses are writing fiction. Creative fiction has long been an underground pursuit
among nurses.

Nursing can view fiction as an opportunity to explore the particular in aesthetic inquiry. Narrative can involve nurses in the
process and product of writing about patients and practice for enhanced personal knowing, without a singular focus on the development of precise methodology.

As process, aesthetic inquiry through narrative has benefits to
offer nurses. Fictional narrative improves recognition of the ambiguity of words and symbols at the heart of nursing practice.
Prolonged contact with fiction (reading or writing) will create enthusiasm for and appreciation of uncertainty.

*Creative literature has a humanizing effect. It helps develop
sensitivity to the complex psychological and physical components of human behavior in health and illness. It wakens us*

*from the numbness that all too frequently accompanies rou-
tine. At the very least, it points to the ambiguity we need to
learn to tolerate in nursing. . . . Creative literature can assist us in gaining this necessary vision. (Bartol, 1986, p. 23)*

This is fundamental for caring in nursing. Caring depends on
caregivers' having knowledge of the general situation and aesthetic knowledge of individuals. Tolerance for ambiguity cannot
be learned in scientific approaches to inquiry; that lesson is contradictory to the intent of science. Aesthetic inquiry, based in
nursing practice and other arts (visual, dramatic, literary), can
teach it.

The stance of the nurse writer in fictional narrative is different
than in other forms of narrative inquiry. Writing requires a prolonged engagement in a frame of mind that constantly and consciously shifts figure–ground relationships. The writer attempts
to maintain an extreme openness and reverence for the particular
because the particular makes more sense within an individual
context. The general, the theoretical, becomes fairly incomprehensible; the writer cannot get a hold on it.

Unlike much scientific inquiry, in aesthetic inquiry the writer
remains fully attached to the phenomenon but not to the product,
which evolves as the writer understands more.

*When you write you lay out a line of words. The line of
words is a miner's pick, a woodcarver's gouge, a surgeon's
probe. . . . You go where the path leads. At the end of the
path, you find a box canyon. You hammer out reports, dis-
patch bulletins. The writing has changed, in your hands,
and in a twinkling, from an expression of your notions to
an epistemological tool. You attend. . . . Courage utterly
opposes the bold hope that this is such fine stuff the work
needs it, or the world. (Dillard, 1989, pp. 3–4)*

Often, what was sought after is completely forgotten and dis-
carded because it is no longer relevant to the search. The real
search is to discover the important questions to address. If writers

do their job earnestly, the questions are rarely the same at the finish of the story.

Future work, similar to a program of scientific inquiry, progresses from the beginning of a work that the writer pares away. A piece may be technically well-written, perhaps the best written, but the writer will often realize that it is peripheral to the meaning of the story. The meaning itself has changed as the story has evolved. The writer is open to unpredictable and, if the writer has integrity, uncontrollable change within the story.

The part you must jettison is not only the best-written part; it is also, oddly, that part which was to have been the very point. It is the original key passage, the passage on which the rest was to hang, and from which you yourself drew the courage to begin. . . . The writer returns to these materials, these passionate subjects, as to unfinished business, for they are his life's work. (Dillard, 1989, pp. 4-5)

The same ambiguity, unclear of purpose beyond that of maintaining connection, distinguishes caring in the best of nursing practice as well as fictional narrative. It is unfolding in purpose and, it is hoped, surprising in outcome. Creative fiction is appropriate to explore the caring situation in the clinical setting because it can retain what is most human—the self, the other, the shared and unique context, feelings as well as thoughts, the smells, and the elusive.

Aesthetic inquiry through narrative is contrary to much of the current research trends in nursing. Nursing is justifying its existence as a scientific profession and is intent on highlighting and supporting efforts that are in concert with that aim. But researchers are struggling to find methods to explore our shared world with patients in ways that reflect the dance of intimacy and distance that is the heart of nursing. Few methods in nursing research are as elastic and contextual as the caring encounter in clinical practice.

Admittedly, aesthetic inquiry will not lead to the clear answers suitable for a profession that is only scientific. If nursing values the privileged ontological stance nurses have with patients, nurses must also value the ambiguous, slippery knowledge of particular patients and individual contexts. Aesthetic inquiry, within what is proposed as a scientific profession, will develop nursing knowledge.

REFERENCES

Abrams, M. (1959). *Mirror and lamp: Romantic theory and the critical tradition.* New York: Oxford University Press.

Bartol, G. (1986). Using the humanities in nursing education. *Nurse Educator, 11*(1), 21-22.

Bartol, G. (1989a). Story in nursing practice. *Nursing and Health Care, 10*(10), 564-565.

Bartol, G. (1989b). Creative literature: An aid to nursing practice. *Nursing and Health Care, 10*(8), 453-457.

Benner, P., & Wrubel, J. (1989). *The primacy of caring: Stress and coping in health and illness.* Menlo Park, CA: Addison-Wesley.

Boykin, A., & Schoenhofer, S. (1991). Story as link between nursing practice, ontology, and epistemology. *Image: The Journal of Nursing Scholarship. 23*(4), 245-248.

Carper, B. (1978). Fundamental patterns of knowing in nursing. *Advances in Nursing Science, 1*(1), 13-23.

Carr, D. (1986). *Time, narrative, and history.* Indianapolis: Indiana University Press.

Dillard, A. (1982a). *Living by fiction.* New York: Harper & Row.

Dillard, A. (1989). *The writing life.* New York: Harper & Row.

Dilthey, W. (1976). The rise of hermeneutics. (T. Hall, Trans.). In P. Connerton (Ed.), *Critical sociology.* New York: Penguin Books. (Original work published 1900)

Gadamer, H.-G. (1989). *Truth and method.* New York: Crossroads Books.

Gadow, G. (1990). *Aesthetics and caring.* Unpublished paper.

Gadow, S. (1990). Response to "Personal knowing: Evolving research and practice." *Scholarly Inquiry for Nursing Practice, 4*(2).

Guba, E. (1990). The alternative paradigm dialog. In E. Guba (Ed.), *The paradigm dialog.* Newbury Park, CA: Sage.

Heidegger, M. (1927). *Being and time* (J. Macquarrie & E. Robinson, Trans.), New York: Harper & Row. (Original work published 1929)

Higgins, D. (1976). *Five traditions of art history, an essay.* New York: Unpublished Editions.

Hillman, J. (1983). *Healing fiction.* Barrytown, NY: Station Hill.

Iser, W. (1978). *The act of reading: A theory of aesthetic response.* Baltimore: The Johns Hopkins University Press.

Jaggar, A. (1989). Love and knowledge: Emotion in feminist epistemology. In A. Jaggar & S. Bordo (Eds.), *Gender/body/knowledge: Feminist reconstructions of being and knowing.* New Brunswick, NJ: Rutgers University Press.

Jakobson, R. (1960). Linguistics and poetry. In T. Seboek (Ed.), *Style and language.* Cambridge: MIT Press.

Knafl, K., & Brietmayer, B. (1991). Triangulation in qualitative research: Concerns and challenges. In J. Morse (Ed.), *Qualitative nursing research: A contemporary dialogue.* Newbury Park, CA: Sage.

Krysl, M. (1991, April). *What is a story good for?* Paper presented at 13th National/International Caring Conference, International Association for Human Caring, University of Rochester, New York.

Le Guin, U. (1989). *Dancing at the edge of the world: Thoughts on words, women, and places.* New York: Harper & Row.

Lincoln, Y., & Guba, E. (1985). *Naturalistic inquiry.* Beverly Hills, CA: Sage.

Livo, N., & Rietz, S. (1986). *Storytelling: Process and practice.* Boulder, CO: Libraries Unlimited.

Long, T. (1986). Narrative unity and clinical judgment. *Theoretical Medicine, 7,* 75-92.

Lopez, B. (1988). *Crossing open ground.* New York: Vintage Books.

Lueders, E. (1989). *Writing natural history: Dialogs with authors.* Salt Lake City: University of Utah Press.

Mink, L. (1978). Narrative form as a cognitive instrument. In R. Canary & H. Kozicki (Eds.). *The writings of history.* Madison: University of Wisconsin Press.

Morse, J. (1991). Qualitative nursing research: A free-for-all? In J. Morse (Ed.), *Qualitative nursing research: A contemporary dialogue.* Newbury Park, CA: Sage.

Nowakowski, J. (1990). A response to so-called training in the so-called alternative paradigm: Reactions to the darker half. In E. Guba (Ed.), *The paradigm dialog.* Newbury Park, CA: Sage.

Polkinghorne, D. (1983). *Methodology for the human sciences: Systems of inquiry.* Albany, NY: SUNY Press.

Polkinghorne, D. (1988). *Narrative knowing and the human sciences.* Albany, NY: SUNY Press.

Preston, J. (1987). Necessary fictions: Healing encounters with a North American saint. *Literature and Medicine, 6,* 42–62.

Reinharz, S. (1990). So-called training in the so-called alternative paradigm. In E. Guba (Ed.), *The paradigm dialog.* Newbury Park, CA: Sage.

Ricouer, P. (1985). *Time and narrative, Vol. 2.* Chicago: University of Chicago Press.

Robinson, I. (1990). Personal narratives, social careers, and medical courses: Analysing life trajectories in autobiographies of people with multiple sclerosis. *Social Science Medicine, 30*(11), 1173–1186.

Sandelowski, M. (1986). The problem of rigor in qualitative research. *Advances in nursing science, 8*(3), 27–37.

Sandelowski, M. (1991). Telling stories: Narrative approaches in qualitative research. *Image: The Journal of Nursing Scholarship, 23*(3), 161–165.

Spence, D. (1982). *Narrative truth and historical truth: Meaning and interpretation in psychoanalysis.* New York: Norton.

Tisdale, S. (1986). *The sorcerer's apprentice: Medical miracles and other disasters.* New York: Holt.

Tisdale, S. (1988). *Harvest moon: Portrait of a nursing home.* Norwalk, CT: Appleton-Century-Crofts.

Vezeau, T. (1993a). Use of narrative in human care inquiry. In D. Gaut (Ed.), *A global agenda for caring.* New York: National League for Nursing.

Vezeau, T. (1993b). Storytelling: A practitioner's tool. *Maternal Child Nursing, 18*(4), 193–196.

Watson, J. (1985). *Nursing: Human science and human care.* Norwalk, CT: Appleton-Century-Crofts.

White, H. (1981). The value of narrativity in the representation of reality. In J. Mitchell (Ed.), *On narrative.* Chicago: University of Chicago Press.

Woolf, V. (1929). *A room of one's own.* New York: Harcourt, Brace, and World.

Younger, J. (1990). Literary works as a mode of knowing. *Image: The Journal of Nursing Scholarship, 22*(1), 39–43.

4

Coming to Moral Consciousness through the Art of Nursing Narratives

M. Katherine Maeve

Since the publication of the writings of Nightingale, the notion of a moral foundation and/or obligation has figured prominently in nursing literature. Nightingale's (1946/1992) legacy was a vision of morality within practice that was very closely associated with religious notions of a god to whom we, as nurses, were duty-bound. This linkage between moral duty and religiosity is troubling, especially given the many divergent spiritual beliefs in our world today. In my experience, when the subject of morality looms in practice, people tend to become somewhat edgy, needing to consider whether they are being good or bad, who might be their judge, and what others may be thinking about them. Morality, or the lack thereof, is worrisome to practitioners. The term moral, or morality, within nursing has not been sufficiently explained and is thus implied to hold a universal understanding within nursing. This, too, is troubling. In her writings about literature and the moral imagination, Nussbaum (1990) noted that "obtuseness is a moral failing; its opposite can be cultivated" (p. 155).

This chapter suggests the cultivation of moral consciousness in practice through the art of nursing narratives, or, as Gadow has suggested, "the moral point of view wants a storied residence" (Gadow, 1993, personal communication). Foundational assumptions will be presented with regard to the terms morality and immorality. The work of Sally Gadow, Jean Watson, Anne Bishop, and John Scudder, Jr., all prominent scholars in nursing literature, will be discussed. Each claims and uses the term moral as foundational to understanding of the philosophy, theory, and/or practice of nursing.

The art form of narratives will be posited as an important way by which to recognize "morally salient images" (Nussbaum, 1990) toward the examination of moral ambiguities in practice. Basic principles of linguistics and philosophy of language will be explored as they specifically relate to languaging and the generation of meaningful narratives. Further, I will propose that the writing of practice narratives is a moral activity by which nurses can explore the art and moral foundation of our practice. Finally, two of my own narratives will be offered. They reflect the good and the bad in my practice as well as the personal beliefs and values that inform my practice.

FOUNDATIONAL UNDERSTANDINGS

Webster's Third New International Dictionary (1986) defines the term moral as relating to principles or considerations of right and wrong action, or right behavior that is sanctioned by, or operating on, one's conscience or ethical judgment. Immorality, then, is defined as being contrary to one's conscience, or a refusal to acknowledge and abide by the boundaries set by convention.

These definitions do not suggest universal understandings within nursing. Reflecting our larger society, nursing is diverse, especially with regard to levels of education and how they impact on the many groups within society to which one can belong. Nursing, too, has its working class, its elite class, and every possibility in between (Maeve, 1994). Although the racial and ethnic mix within nursing continues to favor White women, nursing does include women of color, White men, and men of color. It is suggested that, although many understandings of the term moral would be held in common by the entire group, equally as many, if not more, would not. This diversity is reflected in the nursing literature, which very commonly cites a moral foundation for nursing (Bishop & Scudder, 1987, 1990, 1991; Cooper, 1991; Fry, 1989; Gadow, 1980, 1989a, 1989b; Liaschenko, 1993; Newman, Sime, & Corcoran-Perry, 1991; Nightingale, 1946/1992; Watson, 1985, 1990; Yarling & McElmurry, 1986).

Morality, then requires a clearer explication within the practice of nursing as to the standard by which individual practitioners are to be held accountable. What attributes exist in relation to morality to which we could all agree? The conscience of each individual holds a myriad of possibilities. Yet, realistically, the community of nursing needs to be accountable for the individual practice of its members within a framework that enhances nursing's autonomy, individually and collectively. If we accept a moral accountability for individuals and for the community of nursing, then it becomes crucial for us to examine how we come to know what is immoral.

This issue of immorality is especially important to the community of nursing. Practitioners will find it easier to censor themselves as individuals within their own moral framework. The situation becomes much more complex when we as a community decide what is acceptable and not acceptable from a moral point of view, and then ask for individual and collective accountability to those standards.

This discussion assumes that practitioners have an obligation to articulate their own moral stance to self and others, and to act out this stance in their practice. In other words, practitioners must practice from a base of personal and professional moral integrity. Wheeler and Chinn (1992) would refer to this as praxis, or "values made visible through deliberate action" (p. 2). In line with this thought, Gadow (1993, personal communication) views morality

as values in action, as opposed to ethics, which she views as reflections about values resulting in ethical theory, ethical principles, and ethical critiques.

MORALITY IN THE WORK OF GADOW, WATSON, AND BISHOP AND SCUDDER

Nurse scholars frequently cite the need for theory or philosophically based practice. This section explores how three apparently
similar frameworks would ground the practice of nursing on very
different moral grounds.

Gadow

Gadow's (1980) understandings of the practice of nursing are
founded on what she refers to as existential advocacy. Rather than
theories of nursing, Gadow prefers that nursing be defined and developed from a philosophical stance, which, in Gadow's view, presents an ideal that has more possibility for being fully developed.
Existential advocacy is based on the principle that freedom of self-
determination is a most fundamental and valuable human right.
The nurse, according to Gadow (1980), is in a unique position to
participate with patients as they determine "the unique meaning
which the experience of health, illness, suffering, or dying is to
have for that individual" (p. 81).

In 1982, Gadow used the term moral within the context of the
"best interest" of a patient, noting that moral autonomy was integral to self-determination. Morally autonomous patients could
then engage in a meaningful way in clinical decision making.
Nursing's obligation was to cultivate personal relationships with
patients that would support moral autonomy. Gadow (1989a) described nursing's moral imperative as that of enhancing patient
autonomy through advocacy. Noting that practice is fraught with
moral ambiguity, Gadow offered the "silent" patient as the touch-
stone for exploring nursing's advocacy stance. The truly silent patient has not provided an advance care directive and does not have
relatives, friends, or significant others to offer opinions based on

their experience with this patient. Silent patients' subjectivity is not available to us in conventional ways—through language, for example. Gadow warns against viewing these patients as incompetent, when we only know for certain "that communication—not necessarily competence, is lacking" (1989a, p. 536). Silent patients become our greatest challenge with regard to advocacy, because advocacy requires subjectivity and precludes knowing the body as only object.

In order to view silent patients subjectively, nurses must remain embodied. In this way, over time, "the nurse will slowly sense where the boundary lies between harm and benefit in the patient's world. More than this cannot be known" (Gadow, 1989a, p. 540). Still, Gadow posits, the nurse's translation of this experience, her subjectivity, is the only avenue by which the patient's subjectivity is given voice. Therefore, the embodiment of both patient and nurse remains essential toward the moral commitment to advocacy.

Gadow, in various writings, has defined the care given by nursing as "the alleviation of vulnerability" (Gadow, 1988, p. 7). The alleviation of vulnerability is accomplished through different ways of caring that are, at once, embodied, empathic, and imaginative. The basis of the moral imperative within nursing is the relationship between patient and nurse.

Immorality within Gadow's writings is discerned as the viewing of the body, and patient, as only object. The embodied engagement with patients through the tenets of existential advocacy is seen as a moral activity. The lack of that engagement could also, then, be construed as immoral. And, if our obligation as nurses is to alleviate vulnerability, it could be considered immoral to directly cause, or participate in, the aggravation or increasing of a patient's vulnerability.

Watson

The central theme of all of Watson's writings has been caring. Watson regards what she calls the transpersonal caring relationship as foundational to a caring relationship. A transpersonal caring relationship is characterized as a spiritual union that "occurs between the two persons, where both are capable of transcending self, time, space, and the life history of each other" (1988, p. 66). The transpersonal caring relationship is the moral ideal and essence of nursing. Further, the moral ideal of the transpersonal relationship directly alleviates indignity in humanity and fosters the spiritual evolution of humans individually and collectively. The source of this indignity is never made clear but is sometimes implied to be the result of poor caring practices by other health care professionals. However, if human indignity results from disease, the moral implications are very different.

Like Gadow, Watson urges nurses to direct their interactions with patients toward understanding the meaning of each situation for both participants. This continuity between nurse and patient can result in each creating a life history and is the process of the art of nursing. Watson (1988) noted that she views "this act of transpersonal caring in nursing as a human art, a human science, and a moral ideal of nursing" (p. 68). Because ideals are, by definition, never fully attainable, Watson's moral ideal is wholly unrealizable.

Watson views the soul as the supreme concept within the triad of mind/body/spirit that comprises each human. "[O]ne's soul possesses a body that is not confined by objective space and time" (1988, p. 45). The idea of a soul that can transcend the mind and body through space and time represents a belief system that is similar to Nightingale's (1946/1992). This belief system, however, leaves the body in a kind of "metaphysical isolation" (Jonas, 1966). Watson's framework, therefore, becomes problematic for nurses who have no, or very different, spiritual beliefs.

The basis of nursing's moral obligation in Watson's framework, is the transpersonal relationship with patients, and this relationship is the foundation on which nursing knowledge should be developed; it becomes our substance (1990).

Watson, like Gadow, does not directly address issues of immorality. However, the implied meaning is that if one does not engage in transpersonal relationships as defined in the above discussion, one is not fulfilling nursing's moral imperative and may therefore be practicing immorally. The aggravating or causing of a patient's indignity can also be construed as immoral practice.

Bishop and Scudder

When Bishop and Scudder (1990) first published their philosophy of practice, they noted that the three dominant senses of nursing were (1) practice, (2) moral, and (3) personal. They believe that the primary sense in all health care is not technology or science. Rather, they make a convincing argument that, despite the prevalence of technology and science, the basic nature of care remains moral, particularly in actual practice situations.

More so than Gadow or Watson, Bishop and Scudder have carefully delineated how moral dilemmas are inherent in health care situations. They have identified five general types of moral dilemmas, or tensions, that impact on nursing. The first regards the correctness of particular medical regimes for individual patients. The second is related to the different "intentionalities" that are present in the various professions represented in any health care setting. The third tension exists between the carrying out of objective treatments while attempting to provide intimate, personal care to individuals. Importantly, they have identified a need for practitioners to move back and forth between objectivity and subjectivity, and in this way they differ sharply from Gadow and Watson. The fourth tension exists as nursing attempts to provide specialized input to an interdisciplinary health care team. The fifth tension exists as nurses attempt to develop personal, helping relationships within a bureaucracy that tends not to honor or respect these relationships over time.

These tensions imply the moral dilemmas that present themselves in the everyday practice of nursing. Many of these dilemmas are not solvable; nevertheless, they do exist and must be dealt with because they occur in the real lives of real people, as opposed to viewing them in the abstract.

Bishop and Scudder (1990, 1991) have been very clear that the moral sense of practice is grounded in the notion of "good." Indeed, they noted that nursing has historically been developed from good care in a way that affirms the way as well as the ends. Their moral imperative is of a caring ethic that stresses responsible relationships in which nurses strive for good care through sound, excellent practice. "[S]ince excellent practice fosters human good, the primary moral responsibility of the nurse is excellent practice" (1991, p. 105). Within this framework, a nurse could never be described as very caring and yet incompetent. Caring, in Bishop and Scudder's work, subsumes competency, which includes competence in technology.

Bishop and Scudder differ from Gadow and Watson in that the moral sense that predominates in relationships between nurse and patient is not considered an individual event. Rather, Bishop and Scudder confirm the notion that "excellent practice both shapes and is shaped by other excellent practice" (Maeve, 1994). The moral imperative for Bishop and Scudder includes the notion of critique within the community of nursing toward the moral goal of excellent practice.

Another important difference separating Bishop and Scudder from Gadow and Watson is the expectation that patients are active participants in the moral functions and activities of health care. For instance, patients are expected to be responsible for acknowledging good care they receive as a general human responsibility toward affirming the goodness in others. Nurses, in turn, may help patients identify and articulate their own moral foundational beliefs, thus enabling patients to more fully participate in their health care within an awareness of their own beliefs and values.

Of serious concern are Bishop and Scudder's contentions that nurses are morally obligated to carry out regimes prescribed by physicians, to maintain order in care, and to support policies put forth by the institutions to which they belong. A complete exploration of this puzzling view is beyond the intent and scope of this chapter. However, as an example, Bishop and Scudder describe an occasion when a nurse smuggled in a two-year-old grandchild, against hospital policy, so that a patient could die surrounded by his family. Hutchinson (1990) would refer to this as "responsible subversion," an action most nurses would sanction. However, to explicitly identify morality within practice as upholding institutional policies and at the same time cite morality as a cause for violating those policies puts nurses in an untenable position, further invalidates our power as individuals and as a profession, and seriously impinges on the quest toward excellence in practice.

Notions of immorality are very clear in Bishop and Scudder's work. It is immoral not to give good care; not to use sound practice knowledge; not to care; and not to want to try to be a good nurse. An incompetent nurse practices immorally regardless of how "nice" she might be to the patients in her care. Further, it is considered immoral to not share nursing's responsibility individually and collectively. Paradoxically, however, Bishop and Scudder have also implied that not upholding institutional policies and physicians' expectations is immoral.

Table 1 summarizes the major characteristics of the three frameworks. The common thread among the frameworks is the endorsement of personal relationships as foundational to nursing. The concepts of morality and immorality, while sharing some characteristics, are clearly not the same in each framework. All of these authors acknowledge the practice of nursing as a moral activity and implicitly validate the need to examine practice, individually and collectively, from the perspective of moral intentionality.

These three nursing frameworks, which externally appear to have many similarities, give different direction toward the understanding of moral and/or immoral practice. As previously noted, the concept of morality and immorality in nursing remains to be sufficiently explored.

ART AND NURSING

Undoubtedly, in this anthology devoted to the art of nursing, many understandings of art will be set forth. One aspect assumed in this work is that art reflects human understanding and, in so doing, reflects our morality as well. Art, regardless of form, has traditionally served as a crucible for morality. Art reflects morality inasmuch as it serves to show us what we do not consider moral and validates what we do consider moral. In other words, art has traditionally reflected the moral consciousness of the artist and has informed the moral consciousness of the spectator, observer, or participant.

In a society where art is often an expression of politics, art forms committed to free expression assume even greater meaning. Recorded history is full of accounts of writers, painters, and

Table 1

Theorist(s)/ Philosopher	Aspects of Morality	Aspects of Immorality
Gadow's Framework: Existential Advocacy	1. Moral sense lies in personal relationships as nurses alleviate vulnerability for individual patients.	1. Aggravating or increasing a patient's vulnerability.
	2. Nurses must remain vulnerable to the subjectivity of their patients (embodied engagement).	2. Viewing patients and bodies as objects while remaining in a disembodied state.
	3. Moral autonomy is a basic human right for both nurses and patients.	3. Violating one's moral consciousness, or disabling another's moral autonomy.
Watson's Framework: Nursing as Human Science and Human Care	1. Spiritual unions with patients within transpersonal caring relationships, capable of transcending time and space.	1. Nonrecognition of or disbelief in the spiritual nature of humans, thus precluding the formation of a spiritual union within a transpersonal caring relationship.
	2. Alleviation of human indignity through transpersonal caring.	2. Aggravating or causing indignity to a patient.
Bishop and Scudder's Framework: Nursing as the Practice of Caring	1. Moral imperative of the development of excellent nursing practice, individually and collectively.	1. Incompetence in practice and the tolerance of incompetence in others.
	2. Moral sense of nursing realized through personal relationships aimed toward fostering the well-being of patients through caring.	2. Unwillingness to care.
	3. Nurses' moral obligation to carry out physicians' orders as well as institutional policies.	3. Unwillingness to execute physicians' orders or subversion of institutional policies.

artists who were severely castigated for works that were considered immoral. Grubin (1993), in a film recently shown on public television, detailed how the Nazis used art as a weapon against thought and imagination that did not reflect their particular brand of ideology. Art, in all forms, that represented alternate points of view was branded as degenerate art, or *entartete kunst*. Written art was burned. Art in the form of paintings and sculptures was put on display in a manner that required visitors to the exhibition to understand how art of this kind might cause degeneration of their society, how it might taint their intended purity. The offensive art did not portray life as beautiful and serene; instead, it often portrayed the ugliness and bitterness that are also part of humanity, as well as various abstract interpretations.

There is a lesson here for nursing. Early in my doctoral education, I attended a class that was assigned to read Tisdale's (1986) *The Sorcerer's Apprentice: Medical Miracles and Other Disasters.* Tisdale, a nurse, recounts her life as a bedside nurse, a place I occupied for 17 years of my career. Others in the class, however, who had long left the bedside staff-nurse role, complained that these stories were ugly and bitter, not representative of their reality. In their view, Tisdale was dour and unnecessarily harsh. Yet, I recognized every word, every phrase, for I had lived them all. There is a tendency in nursing to give high regard only to stories that reflect the beauty involved in personal relationships with patients. We prefer beautiful art, beautiful outcomes.

A critique of Tisdale's work is not at issue here; her choice of artistic representation—narrative—is. Tisdale, myself, and others have used narrative as a way to approach an understanding of the complex moral struggles in our practice.

NARRATIVES AND NURSING

Principles of Language and Narratives

Linguists and philosophers of language provide an important backdrop for understanding how narratives can accomplish the goals of reflecting and informing our moral consciousness.

Saussure (1983), who pioneered semiology (the study of signs in social life) in the early 1900s, was the first major linguist of our time. A major premise of Saussure was that language is not created, destroyed, or controlled by any individual or group of individuals. Rather, once language comes in contact with communities or populations at large, language evolves and develops. A person may approach language changes with intentionality, but the way language actually develops is not predetermined by that same intentionality. Language, then, is fortuitous, or without deliberate intention.

Saussure posited that language is composed of linguistic signs, which are comprised of the signified and the signifier, such as the mental image of a table and the actual word table. Scholes (1980) Peirce's argument for another component, the interpretant, existed between the signified and signifier. The interpretant functioned to arrive at the signifier by mediating that process with the speaker's history and background. For instance, when I think of a table, I think of a big round oak table, because that is my referent. I have had a big round oak table in my dinning room all of my life. Therefore, my understanding of table in any context always begins in opposition to my oak table. The importance of this will become apparent shortly.

Smith (1981) designated basic stories from narrative versions of events. Basic stories reflect basic facts that would probably not change much between speakers. Stories become narratives when the stories are retold from particular or partial perspectives. "Narratives are constructed by someone in particular, on some occasion, for some purpose, and in accord with some relevant set of principles" (Smith, 1981, p. 214). For example, the narratives I write are directed toward a particular audience—other nurses—and are based on my knowledge of those nurses and the possible circumstances that will bring them to my narratives. The narratives were conceived by me and were written in a language that was directly impacted on by the feedback of the same audience who had heard me tell the story, before it was collapsed into words on paper.

It therefore becomes impossible to sort out any single function of any single narrative. The range of possible narrative transactions and interests is so wide among humans that we must acknowledge a multiplicity of functions present in narratives in general and in any particular narrative.

Narratives, then, are constantly in process, and the process is different for each individual exposed to a narrative. Even narratives that have been written and copyrighted remain process among the readers and for the narrator because the nature of narratives is narration, or an oral tradition. For instance, when I think of a table, my mind begins with the mental concept of a round oak table; however, because my life experience has shown me many varieties of tables, my mental concept of a table is infinitely more complex than when I was a little girl. I have many images of tables against which to compare the construct of table. Narratives must be viewed, then, as intimate reflections of their writers—reflections that may never be fully understood.

Narratives, as noted above, represent the telling and retelling of basic stories (Smith, 1981). For both the narrator and the listener, each retelling is impacted on by the previous telling. Narratives, then, are abstracted personal versions of basic stories.

Another important feature of narratives involves what linguists refer to as case grammar. Donnelly (1993) stated that case grammar is a model that reflects the way the human mind actually processes text. She defined case grammar as consisting of a sentence structure that contains two parts: (1) a verb, or action, and (2) the arguments, which consist of noun phrases. Each noun phrase has a function or role: an agent is always identified, or someone (or something) with a clear function is always integral to the verb or action.

When agency in a sentence or text is obscured, responsibility is also obscured. For example, Donnelly cited a portion of text written by the pilot who dropped the nuclear bomb on Nagasaki during World War II (1993, pp. 59-60):

But at this moment no one yet knows which one of the several cities chosen as targets is to be annihilated. The final choice lies with destiny. The winds over Japan will make the decision. If they carry heavy clouds over our primary target, that city will be saved, at least for the time being . . . . The winds of destiny seemed to favor certain Japanese cities that must remain nameless. We circled about them again and again and found no opening in the thick umbrella of clouds that covered them. Destiny chose Nagasaki as the ultimate target.

The pilot's account has obscured his responsibility by designating "destiny" and "the winds" as the responsible agents in this event. "Responsibility is obscured to protect the agent immediately responsible for the bombing—the bombers themselves" (Donnelly, 1993, p. 60). Donnelly (1993) argued strongly that the objective language traditionally used in scientific texts creates the illusion that the researcher or agent is so removed as to be objective, but is equally removed from responsibility. Rather, Donnelly urged writers in all mediums to ". . . claim credit for what you have written. You should never be afraid to be authoritative; you are always the authority for your own text" (1993, p. 64).

Donnelly's work is important here for several reasons. The very nature of narratives represents the agent clearly, for the reasons Donnelly identifies. Narratives are the result of explorations of the personal; and, in our language, personal consists of gender. Drawing on the work of Saussure, Donnelly (1993) noted the failure of those who would posit a genderless language using genderless pronouns. In our language, we recognize "he" and "she," not "s/he" or "he/she." Donnelly encouraged the liberal use of either pronoun, depending on the view and choice of the writer.

Of even greater importance is the call for nurses to assume agency in all their writings. For instance, how would direct patient care change if we assumed responsibility for our actions by identifying ourselves as the responsible agents? As an example, consider two fictitious chart entries:

1. *Patient complains of abdominal pain. As patient had Demerol only two hours earlier, explained that he could not receive another dose for two more hours.*

2. Donald is asking for more Demerol. I told him he had to wait two more hours because he can only have one dose every four hours.

Both entries reflect the same situation inasmuch as they are abiding by an impersonal, nameless authority. However, the nurse in the second example seems lacking, but only because she has identified herself as a real human being who has chosen not to pursue the matter further for a real person named Donald. In the first example, which I believe is typical charting, the onus for the nurse to react is missing—the glaring personal responsibility to acknowledge and act to alleviate Donald's pain. The nurse in the second example acknowledges Donald's pain, but clearly on a personal level is refusing to take a proactive stance for Donald.

In summary, art in narrative, along with principles of linguistics, represents valuable insights into the exploration of the personal and of morality in practice. Although the actual practice of nursing in time and space is our act of art, that art can be eloquently portrayed in our narratives of practice. As the stories of our practice are told, retold, and retold again, they become our personal practice narratives. The different versions of narratives are not predictable for any individual; they all depend on what the individual is reflecting them from—her own life experience down to the minutest detail. The call for responsibility inherent in the process of creating these narratives is another call for the same responsibility to be acknowledged during the original events. The concept of "narrative charting" needs to be revisited.

NARRATIVES

Two of my own narratives follow. The first, "Mary," was the first narrative I put down on paper. It is easy for me to allow others to read this; the reasons will become obvious. The second narrative, "The Death of Ed," is a different matter altogether. Gadow (1993, personal communication) suggests that morality in nursing is respect and/or regard for "particularity." Each of these narratives represents the cultivation and expression of my particularity, with its passions and its prejudices.

Mary

Mary sits quietly, sternly, yet peacefully in this ICU bed. Her chest bears the scar of surgery on her heart the year before. Her face bears the scars of her past, bittersweet scars uniquely common to women. And, Mary is a woman of 92 years.

In this time and space, Mary's gallbladder is betraying her. Betraying to me, but merely another of life's annoyances to Mary. But, betrayal or annoyance, Mary will not survive without surgery, and may die because of it.

Mary commands me. As I race to complete pre-surgery rituals, Mary instructs me as to the singular order in which she wishes to see her family—one at a time in ascending order of importance to her. The oldest grandson, 16, is next to last. A big hulking boy, he lingers at the door, clearly afraid to enter. She bids him come. He begins a step but stops to hide his face and cry. Mary opens her arms to him and bids him come and lay his head in this grandma's lap. "If a boy can't cry for his Grandma, who can he cry for?" she tells him. He quietly sobs into her blankets and she strokes his hair. Mary tells him the story of her love for him—when he was born, how proud she has been of him as he has grown. "Always know that I loved you, and I know you have loved me. I've had a good life, all the better for you. Now go, be strong and send your mother in." My rituals have stopped in respect. I lower my gaze in the presence of the Goddess.

Mary's rituals are over. The last of mine is to place a tube through Mary's nose into her stomach, so those juices that can't get through to the intestines won't complicate anesthesia. Mary expresses annoyance and acceptance of this uncomfortable "hose." I, too, feel annoyed at having to slide the hose through her nose, but know it is necessary.

Something goes wrong. Mary necessarily chokes and coughs when the tube slides down the back of her throat.

Mary's heart stops its once effective beats and begins to quiver. Mary is dying. I did it.

The ultimate ICU ritual begins. A "code" is called and a new rhythm takes over. I push on Mary's chest and tell her I'm sorry. As I push drugs into her IV line, I tell her it's not time. They indicate I should electro-shock her heart with the paddles, and I hesitate. I know it hurts, I know it burns the flesh, yet I know it works. The paddles are charged, no one else is in a position to hold the paddles on Mary's chest, no one else can push the red buttons and deliver the shock. "Mary, I'm sorry, I don't want to, I have to," and I do. I cry, begging Mary to live, it's not time, I know it's not time. They tell me to do it again. I deliver my apologetic entreaty and zap Mary again. (Only later do I perceive the peculiar glances others have given me while I quietly, yet plaintively plead with Mary.)

The Goddess finally answers. Mary's heart begins a normal rhythm. She breathes, but her eyes are closed, she is silent.

Everyone leaves the room. Some to care for others, some to inform the family what has happened. I automatically begin the "after-the-code-cleanup" ritual. My hands and legs do the work without my conscious instruction, as the very wholeness that is me wants Mary to live—for her and for me. At once, I retrace my steps in placing the tube, looking for blame, while I silently chant my mantra-like desire for Mary to live.

As I have looked away, in rhythm with my own ritual, I turn to see Mary smiling at me. Her gaze is direct and compelling. Mary opens her arms and bids me come. She pulls me down to her and kisses me hard, on my mouth. "I heard you tell me to live, you sweet child." I dissolve into Mary's lap of tears and tell her how sorry I am, maybe I did something wrong. Mary hushes me, strokes my head. Mary absolves me of guilt. Mary says I'm a good nurse. Mary says I'm a good woman.

Mary is the Goddess. (Maeve, 1989).

The Death of Ed

For the last two weeks I have taken care of the same three patients in this ICU. None of them know where they are and sometimes don't even know who they are. My nerves are completely frazzled. One, a truck driver in an accident, is wearing a newly placed halo traction and very much needs to lie still. However, he is unaware of his precarious position and is very angry and resistant. He wants out and keeps trying to get loose of everything so he can bolt. Obviously, however, he can't bolt and sees me and the other nurses as bitches from the hell we've put him in, and continually yells his insults at us. The second, a 72-year-old homeless man who has had a severe heart attack, also doesn't want to be here, wherever "here" is, and likes to pass stool in the bed and then throw it at us. The third patient is my most trying burden. Charlie is 64 and was originally admitted to rule out an myocardial infarction. Initially, he did well, and was well enough to transfer to the transitional care unit. However, it now appears he has precipitated Alzheimer's disease and has been wild.

Charlie has the strength of a teenager and is continually straining at his restraints. Regardless of our efforts, he still manages to kick at me, tries to grab me, he spits at me and tries to hit me with his head. Yesterday, he bit a nurse so severely she required stitches. At the beginning of all this, he jumped out of his bed and hit his wife so hard across the face that she fell to the floor. Over time, she has acknowledged that this is normal behavior for him, she has been a beaten wife for the entire 10 years of their marriage. What is unusual, she says, is that he keeps mistaking her for his first wife.

I have tried everything I know to try. I've tried to keep the lighting so that it mimics night and day. I've tried to keep equipment noise down in his cubicle. I've tried reality orientation so often, I'm starting to confuse myself about what is real. I've tried chatting, I've tried pleading, I've tried ignoring him. I've cajoled some of the male staff into sitting in his room from time to time to talk with him and provide some male companionship. I've eaten my meals in the room with him during his meal time.

Charlie's doctor swoops in once a day and complains that we are keeping his wonderful patient restrained. Don't we know this is a fine upstanding member of the community? Frankly, I don't. Because, over time, I have come to see that Charlie is as he is now—an abusive, violent, nasty man.

Charlie's wife has watched our impatience and resentment of her husband with interest. She confides in me that she has no intention of being in their house if and when he is ever discharged. "I was so scared at first, but these weeks without him have been so peaceful. My children want me to stay with them rather than go back to all of that" she tells me. I squeeze her hand and wish that I, too, did not have to have Charlie in my life.

Before I leave today, however, I have been commanded to get Charlie out of bed and walked around the unit. I get all of my male staff together, carefully untie him, and start the much assisted walking. Charlie is being very cooperative and seems happy to be out of the room. He turns to my friend Steve and quickly bends over to bite his hand. We all jump and I lightly slap Charlie's shoulder and sternly tell him "You may not bite anyone, Charlie." Family members of a newly admitted patient look at us with horror and dread. I don't have a clue what I should do at this point and simply give up and tell them to put him back and retie him.

That brief foray into the hall has everyone in an uproar. I shut the door in Charlie's room so I can cry and get this room cleaned up. Charlie asks me why I'm crying, and I tell him. He nods his head in complete confusion, as always, but closes his eyes for a time. And, then again, he starts becoming agitated shouting at me to "get the door." So, I open the door and tell Charlie that it is open now. "Not that door, stupid, the back door!" "This is the only door I see, Charlie, and it's open; now please be quiet." "You stupid bitch, Ed is at the door!" "Ed couldn't be at the door, Charlie." "Why the hell not?" "Because Ed is dead." "He is?" "Yes, he is." Charlie's

*whole demeanor changes and he asks me when did he die?
"Oh, about a year ago." "Well, I'll be damned."*

*And, for the first time in my experience of Charlie, he lays
back and sleeps for two straight hours. I'm not ashamed,
only relieved. When I arrive home, I immediately call in sick
for the next day because I am sick—I have hate in my heart.
I am wounded. Enough is enough. (Maeve, 1993).*

CONCLUSION

Any moral insights or knowledge in the preceding narratives, as
Cooper (1991) suggests, will be left for you to decide. Nussbaum
(1990) noted that "moral knowledge is not simply an intellectual
grasp of propositions; it is a complex, concrete reality in a highly
lucid and richly responsive way" (p. 152). You are invited to examine the various aspects of these narratives in light of your own experience and practice, and I hope that you are able to judge the
exemplars of my practice with kindness. I also invite you to examine the narratives in light of the previous discussion of morality
and immorality in the work of Gadow, Watson, and Bishop and
Scudder, and the different standards to which I would be held accountable. Our moral struggles are contextual and complex, and
they do not lend themselves to easy answers.

Given the complex nature of practice, we must remain cogni-
zant of the need to encourage creativity and artfulness in other
nurses and not just expect and reward conformity. We cannot remain detached from our moral conflicts for fear of being judged;
rather, we must create a safe atmosphere in which nurses can
share these conflicts and burdens in a way that will support and
nurture nurses individually and collectively. Our art, like the art
tortured into submission by the Nazis, is not always beautiful and
sweet. Our art sometimes is ugly, sometimes stinks, sometimes is
glorious, but always reflects our values, understandings, and ambiguities. Our art can reflect the horror of immoral acts, and our art
can reflect the morality of our choices, our responsibility.

Narratives are a natural way for nurses to explore their practice while retaining their agency and responsibility. Street (1990)

challenged us to write of practice, noting that, if we do, we can then "begin to move from passivity in the face of authority, pessimism in the face of challenges and dilemmas, and vicitimisation of their peers" (p. 30). As previously noted, art in our society is often an expression of the political. Our narratives, therefore, because they express our art, hold the potential for power and change.

The development of moral knowledge, identified as such, is vital to the development of the profession of nursing. That knowledge is in our stories, waiting only to be retold, discovered, and rediscovered.

REFERENCES

Bishop, A., & Scudder, J. (1987). Nursing ethics in an age of controversy. *Advances in Nursing Science, 9*(3), 34-43.

Bishop, A., & Scudder, J. (1990). *The practical, moral and personal sense of nursing.* New York: SUNY Press.

Bishop, A., & Scudder, J. (1991). *Nursing: The practice of caring.* New York: National League for Nursing.

Cooper, M. (1991). Principle-oriented ethics and the ethic of care: A creative tension. *Advances in Nursing Science, 14*(2), 22-31.

Donnelly, C. (1993). *Linguistics for writers.* New York: SUNY Press.

Fry, S. (1989). Toward a theory of nursing ethics. *Advances in Nursing Science, 11*,(4), 9-22.

Gadow, S. (1980). Existential advocacy: Philosophical foundation of nursing. In S. Spicker & S. Gadow (Eds.), *Nursing: Images and ideals* (pp. 79-101). New York: Springer.

Gadow, S. (1982). Allocating autonomy: Can patients and practitioners share? In R. A. Wright (Ed.), *Human values in health care* (pp. 235-245). New York: McGraw-Hill.

Gadow, S. (1988). Covenant without cure: Letting go and holding on in chronic illness. In J. Watson & M. Ray (Eds.), *The ethics of care and the ethics of cure: Synthesis in chronicity* (pp. 5-14). New York: National League for Nursing.

Gadow, S. (1989a). Clinical subjectivity: Advocacy with silent patients. *Nursing Clinics of North America, 24*(2), 535-541.

Gadow, S. (1989b). Remembered in the body: Pain and moral uncertainty. In L. Kliever (Ed.), *Dax's case: Essays in medical ethics and human meaning* (pp. 151-167). Dallas: Southern Methodist University Press.

Grubin, D. (Producer and Director) (1993). *Degenerate art* (film). In association with the Los Angeles City Museum of Art. Los Angeles: David Grubin Productions.

Hutchinson, S. (1990). Responsible subversion: A study of rule bending among nurses. *Scholarly Inquiry for Nursing Practice, 4*(1), 3-17.

Jonas, H. (1966). *The phenomenon of life: Toward a philosophical biology*. Chicago: University of Chicago Press.

Liaschenko, J. (1993). Feminist ethics and cultural ethos: Revisiting a nursing debate. *Advances in Nursing Science, 15*(4), 71-81.

Maeve, M. K. (1989). *Mary*. Unpublished story, Denver, Co.

Maeve, M. K. (1993, March). *The carrier bag theory of nursing practice*. Paper presented to conference on Critical and Feminist Theory in Nursing, Atlanta, GA.

Maeve, M. K. (1993). *The death of Ed*. Unpublished story, Denver, Co.

Maeve, M. K. (1994). The carrier bag theory of nursing practice. *Advances in Nursing Science, 16*(4), in press.

Newman, M., Sime, A. M., & Corcoran-Perry, S. (1991). The focus of the discipline of nursing. *Advances in Nursing Science, 14*(1), 1-6.

Nightingale, F. (1992). *Notes on nursing*. Commemorative Edition, B. Barnum (Ed.). Philadelphia: Lippincott. (Updating 1946 edition)

Nussbaum, M. (1990). *Love's knowledge: Essays on philosophy and literature*. New York: Oxford University Press.

Saussure, F. (1988). *Course in general linguistics* (R. Harris, Trans.). LaSalle, IL: Open Court Publishing Co.

Scholes, R. (1981). Afterthoughts on narrative: Language, narrative, and anti-narrative. In W.J.T. Mitchell (Ed.) *On narrative* (pp. 200-208). Chicago: University of Chicago Press.

Smith, B. H. (1981). Afterthoughts on narrative: Narrative versions, narrative theories. In W.J.T. Mitchell (Ed.) *On narrative* (pp. 209-232). Chicago: University of Chicago Press.

Street, A. (1990). *Nursing practice—High, hard ground, messy swamps and the pathways in between*. Geelong, Victoria, Australia: Deakin University Press.

Tisdale, S. (1986). *The sorcerer's apprentice: Medical miracles and other disasters*. New York: Henry Holt and Company.

Watson, J. (1985). *Nursing: The philosophy and science of caring*. Boulder: Colorado Associated University Press.

Watson, J. (1988). *Nursing: Human science and human care.* New York: National League for Nursing.

Watson, J. (1990). Caring knowledge and informed moral passion. *Advances in Nursing Science, 13*(1), 15-24.

Wheeler, C. E., & Chinn, P. (1991). *Peace & power: A handbook of feminist process (3rd ed.).* New York: National League for Nursing.

Yarling, R., & McElmurry, B. (1986). The moral foundation of nursing. *Advances in Nursing Science, 8*(2), 63-73.

5

The Gift of Self:
A Paradigm for Originating
Nursing as Art

Cathy Appleton

*T*his research study explicates nursing as an art from the perspective of its meaning for the patient and nurse. Five distinct meta-themes express the experience of the art of nursing:

1. Being there;
2. Being-with each other in understanding;
3. Creating opportunities for fullness of being;
4. A transcendent togetherness;
5. A context of caring. (Appleton, 1993).

In caring, nurses originate nursing with the patient and cocreate a unique way of helping characterized as liberating and emancipatory (Appleton, 1991).

From descriptions of patients' and nurses' experiences, a paradigm of originating nursing and cocreating it as art is revealed. This paradigm (1) challenges the singular biomedical approach to health care by offering knowledge of the art of nursing and (2) provides an empirical base from which innovative *models of nursing* can evolve. By explicating nursing as an original experience, the art of nursing reconciles the conceptual question about caring and well-being and grounds these concepts in a practice of nursing as art.

MODERN SCIENCE, THEORETICAL TRANSITIONS, AND NURSING INQUIRY

Study of the art of nursing has empirical value for the profession and is consistent with historical and contemporary views of nursing. Conceptualizations found in the literature authored by early leaders reveal a personal, professional approach to comprehending the nature of nursing as art (Nightingale, 1969; Nutting & Dock, 1912; Stewart, 1929). For example, Nightingale's (1969) description of nursing as fine art assigned a universal idea about the qualities of art in nursing.

Study of the nature of the art of nursing requires a philosophical perspective and methodological approach capable of explicating its complex nature within the context of a system of health care. Our literature reveals a lack of research on the experience of the art of nursing, yet theories of nursing abound with ideas about nursing as art. Is the absence of knowledge about the origins and creation of nursing as art related to the profession's scientific heritage and research tradition?

Schon (1984) suggested that we need inquiry into the epistemology of practice. Traditional professional knowledge comes from a model of Technical Rationality that has dominated thinking about professions and has shaped professional practice into "instrumental problem solving made rigorous by the application of scientific theory and technique" (p. 21). Questioning this model, Schon recommended that we search for what constitutes professional practice or knowledge-in-action.

By introducing the idea of reflective practice, he argued that traditional epistemology has left many practitioners in a dilemma of "rigor or relevance" (p. 44). All to frequently, professionals cut the practice situation to fit professional knowledge. This, he believed, contributed to a "crisis of confidence" in professionals: practice situations are always uncertain, complex, unique, and unstable. Schon stated that what professionals need is a science of design, "an epistemology of practice implicit in the artistic, intuitive processes which some practitioners do bring to situations of uncertainty, instability, uniqueness, and value conflict." (p. 49)

As postmodernism provides an opportunity for this line of questioning, the profession of nursing moves toward grounding knowledge in a paradigm of holism and transformation. Consistent with perspectives of art, a paradigm of holism and transformation opens inquiry into nursing as a practice and allows for discovery of its art.

For example, phenomenology as philosophy not only provides a framework for understanding people as unique human beings in relationship to one another and their world, but also offers an approach to science that considers the unique meanings that cohere with diverse experience (Husserl, 1970; van Manen, 1984, 1990), a compatible perspective with notions of holism, transformation, and uncovering a practice epistemology.

Through direct inquiry into the experience of the art of nursing, knowledge that distinguishes nursing as art emerged. The research findings provide a description of an epistemology of knowledge-in-action (Schon, 1984) that portrays the practice of nursing as art. From a phenomenological philosophic perspective of science, the art of nursing reflects the interconnection of an ontology, epistemology, and axiology base experienced as a praxis gestalt.

A PROCESS OF INQUIRY: DISCOVERING THE MEANING OF THE ART OF NURSING

Phenomenology, the basis of this research on the art of nursing, is one of the most valuable philosophical approaches to inquiry for explicating meaning and describing experience. According to

Reeder (1988), originary experience as described by Husserl (1970) allows for access to the structures of experience that constitute consciousness. When an experience is known in terms of how it is constituted and the meaning it holds for the knower, then understanding is fulfilled concerning that phenomenon. Phenomenological inquiry accepts the descriptions of lived experience as the credible source of meaning in the world.

Ray (1990) stated that "experience is known through existential (being-in-the-world) and hermeneutic (interpretive) thought with which phenomenology as a method concerns itself" (p. 176). By understanding the essence revealed in descriptions of the everyday lived experience, we come to know the meaning of an experience. According to Ray (1991), a phenomenological–hermeneutic approach to inquiry explores the empirical experience in which the complex artistic processes of nursing are lived through the interaction of nurse and patient (Ray, 1991).

Ray's (1990, 1991) ideas derive primarily from Husserl (1970), van Manen (1984, 1990), Reeder (1987, 1988), and other human science philosophers and researchers. The method developed by Ray is a reflective and intuitive approach among the following activities that form the process of inquiry used in this study:

1. Explicating the intentionality of the inner being of the researcher;
2. Engaging in a dialog (with participants) describing the art of nursing;
3. Reflecting on the phenomenon and transforming the transcriptions;
4. Moving phenomenological theorizing to a theory of the meaning of the phenomenon;
5. Reviewing written texts and examining similarities and differences as they relate to the research findings.

According to Ray (1991), presuppositions or the intentionality of the inner being of the researcher became known through attentive reflection on one's beliefs and knowledge. The researcher deliberately made known the empirical basis that was bracketed and held in abeyance during the early phases of phenomenological inquiry.

Engaging in a dialog with participants describing the art of nursing began with selecting participants who stated that they experienced nursing as art. Volunteers who responded to announcements posted at outpatient clinics and centers of nursing or who heard about the study through word of mouth were selected based on their experience and their willingness to describe it. The study began with an indeterminate sample size of participants. Data collection began and continued until saturation was reached, that is, when the researcher believed the description of the phenomenon was essentially the same with the exception of some specific details (Glasser & Strauss, 1967).

Six participants who were patients volunteered to participate. The researcher asked each participant to identify the nurse with whom the patient experienced the art of nursing. Five nurses were identified by the participants, and each nurse confirmed the experience of nursing as art. The six patients and five nurses consented in writing to participate in the study. When the eleven individual interviews were completed, each patient was joined by the nurse with whom the patient had experienced the art of nursing, and together they described the experience they had shared. A total of seventeen interviews comprised the basis of the descriptive narrative collected for this study.

Phenomenological reflecting and transforming, a process in the flow of analysis, began with the first encounter with the transcribed data. This encounter involved bracketed reflection. The language in the texts (transcription) was studied and the descriptive experiences were highlighted. Particular emphasis was placed on illuminating the language and structure of the participants' experiences. Immanent themes (linguistic dimensions) were revealed through interpretive reflecting (hermeneutical thinking or unbracketed reflecting). Metathemes, or the more global abstractions of the themes, occurred through a process of phenomenological writing and transforming.

Phenomenological reducing or intuiting, a process of turning to the nature of the transcendental meaning, then occurred. Grasping the unity of meaning as a direct, unmediated apprehension of the whole experience was reached by a "coming together" of the variations and similarities of the experience (Ray, 1991, p. 186). The meaning of the art of nursing that emerged from the study comprised the descriptions, themes, metathemes, unity of meaning, and metaphor, providing a form of knowledge in action or a paradigm of nursing practiced as art.

Reflection on existing research and theoretical work revealed similarities to and differences from the phenomenologically analyzed data. The meaning of the art of nursing gave rise to its value in relation to existing scholarly work.

Credibility and significance are viewed from a phenomenological philosophical perspective of scientific inquiry. The quality of evidence reflects how well the study permeated and portrayed the lived experience described by the participants who know the art of nursing.

A PARADIGM FOR ORIGINATING NURSING

The method of this study evoked and constituted the meaning of the art of nursing experienced by participants who engage in nursing as art. Through a process of interpretive reflecting, the themes that expressed the participants' language of experience were transformed into the metathemes, noted earlier, that provide a paradigm for originating nursing. Expressing the art of nursing, these metathemes—being there, being-with each other in understanding, creating opportunities for fullness of being, a transcendent togetherness, and a context of caring—distinctly illustrate what the patient and the nurse experienced (Appleton, 1993). In the following sections, the meaning of the art of nursing is explored for each of the metathemes that emerged. Each recreated the values, qualities and processes found to constitute nursing as an art. Pseudonyms are given to facilitate the narratives.

Being There

According to the participants' descriptions the person of the nurse and of the patient is central to the art of nursing. The nurse practices nursing from a humanistic perspective of the patient as a whole person, feels compassion for the person in need, and becomes personally involved in helping through caring.

Nursing originates with the patient, who is the primary focus of the nurse. The patient, a person within the context of an entire life, is central to the nurse and is the most important focus of nursing. The nurse perceives the patient as unique, a person of dignity and worth. Describing this perspective, Mary (the patient) commented on the nurse's approach to her and provided an example of the nurse's perspective in action:

> *Marilyn [the nurse] just cares so much more about you than what you weigh at the time, where your fundus is, or how big the baby is. She asks, "How are you feeling?" and, "How are things going at home?" bringing your whole life together as a circle and not just working on one segment. Marilyn sees you as a whole, not just your physical well-being.*

Patients state that this perspective "makes a difference in the experience of nursing." They say it contributes to "more of a personal connection" for them with the nurse. The nurse's sensitivity to the importance of the whole person within the context of an entire life offers distinct grounding for nursing and for the nurse who recognizes what the patient needs and responds in a way experienced as helpful. According to the participants, recognizing the patient's needs from this holistic perspective facilitates the nurse's compassionate response and generates a desire to become personally involved in caring. One patient states:

> *On the visits she would always have compassion. She would always ask, "What hurts?" or "How do you feel?" It made me feel like someone cared, that she wasn't just here doing a job. She got into what she did. She enjoyed it and I didn't feel alone.*

By becoming personally involved, the nurse comes to know the patient as a person. From this personal approach of the nurse, a distinct involvement experienced as sincere, genuine concern transpires. The nurse communicates openly and honestly. Patients state that this demonstrates respect for them as people and indicates the nurse is sincerely committed and willing to help. Mary, a patient, described her experience with Trudy, a nurse, whose honesty and concern for Mary signaled a commitment to become involved in helping in ways Mary wanted to be helped. Trudy, who was not Mary's nurse, unexpectedly was called to assist Mary in giving birth:

> *All of a sudden two of us were pushing at the same time and [my] midwife couldn't help us both. So Trudy [midwife] came in and she told me very honestly, "Well, I have to tell you I haven't read your birth plan." Gretchen [Mary's primary nurse] had read it and knew everything in it, so she told Trudy. I'm glad Trudy told me instead of trying to pry what she wanted out of me. I'm glad she just came out and said, "I just didn't get a chance to read it and I know it's important to you and I want to know what you want."*

The nurse's concern for the patient, expressed as truth-telling, characterizes the involvement of the nurse in helping and establishes the nature of caring in the practice of nursing as art. The nurse and patient deliberately work at knowing each other, feel comfortable relating personally, and cultivate a deep person-to-person relationship. Authentic concern and personal involvement in helping describe the way the nurse is being there in caring for patients.

Equally significant is the patient's way of being there in relation to the nurse. The patient—described as centering on needing care, feeling vulnerable in a time of need, and personally involved in wanting help through the caring of the nurse—seeks help and wants the nurse's caring to be kind, considerate, and pleasant. In the art of nursing, the expression of kindness and consideration diminishes interpersonal strangeness and makes comfort possible for the patient who, in a time of need, feels vulnerable. Patients describe feeling nervous, tense, scared, worried, and sometimes out of control. Uncertainty becomes magnified in times of transition, when patients feel especially vulnerable. Sally, a patient, related feeling comfortable with the nurse:

> *[W]ith Audrey [the nurse] I wasn't really scared because I knew it was going to be okay. I mean, of course you're scared to a point because you are in such a vulnerable position and anything can happen. But it wasn't like when I was in the hospital with the first one. I really didn't have the worries, frustrations, and anxiety running through me like I had with the first one in the hospital.*

Patients want their feelings of nervousness, tension, fear, and uncertainty acknowledged. Nurses who acknowledge the patients' vulnerability and realize its potential for self-fulfillment are received by patients and given permission to care. Nurses who commit to patients in this manner create an experience of nursing that patients describe as "safe." These nurses personalize caring to the need of the patients, and the patients' feeling of vulnerability (uncomfortable and uncertain) becomes endurable:

> *I saw two totally different experiences. It made me appreciate what nursing could be and how it could be an art instead of just a day-to-day job. I found there are people [referring to Marilyn, the nurse] out there that really care about you and feel that nursing is like their calling, almost like a religious thing. The nurse that I had was just so close and she cared about everything. It's like she just cares so much more about you.*

In seeking the assistance nurses offer, patients expect competent nursing care. Patients desire devotion from the nurse: for them, it demonstrates a nurse's professional commitment in contrast to a nurse who considers nursing "just a job."

In the nurse's way of being there, an open and honest relating expresses genuine concern and communicates the personal involvement of helping in caring. The commitment and devotion of the nurse create a connection that eventually becomes more than a working relationship for the patient and nurse. Trust begins to develop when the nurse deliberately affirms patients by acknowledging their experience and needs. Feeling comfortable and free to express themselves, the nurse and patient begin to come to know one another and develop a mutual understanding.

Being-With Each Other in Understanding

In being-with each other, participants describe a shift away from the distinct way they (the nurse and patient) entered the experience of nursing and toward becoming closely involved or relating intimately. In the first metatheme, the nurse and patient enter the experience of nursing and the nurse is there. In developing understanding, the nurse becomes intimately involved with the patient, knows the patient uniquely by recognizing the meaning the experience holds, and is able to connect with the person of the patient in a relationship that is necessary for helping.

By developing a connection with patients, the nurse intends to come to know what the experience is like for them. "Empathizing" and "intuiting" describe the nurse who establishes a correspondence between the nature of the needs of patients and being-with them in ways characterized as helping. The nurse's intent to know patients and to explicate their wishes transpires in empathizing and intuiting. Intrinsic to the art of nursing, empathic and intuitive knowledge empowers a relationship between nurse and patient. By empathically and intuitively knowing, the nurse is able to individualize caring in a way the patient experiences as helpful:

She sort of knew when we needed things. It was a premonition that you needed something, that you needed somebody to come up to you and say, this will all be over. She is there when you need her. It just seems sort of strange how she pops in all of a sudden the moment you had just thought, I really need somebody in here or I'm going to lose it because I feel strange. I need something. She kept coming in and she seemed to know. She knew when I needed to talk to someone in between contractions.

In empathy, nurses acknowledge the meaning of the experience for patients. Empathy constitutes skill in nursing and enlarges the bond between nurse and patient. The ability to sense and feel what the patient experiences enhances intimacy, and the nurse intuitively comes to know the patient and what matters more deeply. Participants state that intuition entails knowing something "unexplainable" yet present to the nurse. "Having another sense" about the rightness of an experience for the patient speaks of the importance both empathy and intuition hold as knowledge-in-action.

As the relationship deepens, the nurse and patient develop a bond of friendship. The nurse safeguards the patient's integrity and creates nursing consistent with the choices the patient makes. By sharing experiences with each other, nurses respect the wishes of patients and deliberatively act to honor these wishes and maintain patients' integrity in the process. Patients know the nurse keeps their welfare and best interest at heart. This expression of the nurse's caring entails a nonintrusive and noninvasive practice, thereby recognizing the patient's responsibility to make choices and determine quality of life.

When nurses trust their knowledge, ability, and skill, they are empowered to trust patients. In turn, patients trust that their vulnerability in a time of need and transition will not place them at a disadvantage. The relationship that develops from trust speaks of the nurse's belief in the patient's competency to achieve the identified aim and of the patient's belief in the nurse's ability to help. Mary described the trust she experienced with the nurses:

> *You call them in the middle of the night and they are dead asleep and they say, "Listen, don't worry that's what we're here for" or they just explain what's going on or they will say, "I'm here for you." The way they tell you, you believe them. The trust is built through your whole relationship. You have this experience with them for nine months and you gain this trust and this caring, this loving feeling for them that they're going to take care of you.*

Reliance on the nurse, the patient, and the process of nursing is evidence of the completeness of trusting that exists in the art of nursing. This trust centers on the process of living one's meaning of life in the moment and emerges as faith in the future. Based on the nurse's commitment to patients and the patients' commitment to care for themselves, a bond forms and the relationship deepens to become one of a mutually shared experience grounded in trust and respect:

Audrey [the nurse] was right there at the time, but without interfering, without getting into my personal space between myself and my husband. She looked after every need I had but she wasn't pushy about it. She really respected my wishes that I put in my birth plan.

Originating nursing as an art speaks to the importance of this distinct relationship nurses have with patients. It requires opportunity and time to develop and strengthen—spending time in coming to know the person who is a patient, and taking the time needed by patients to express caring for them. When nurses "give their best," as demonstrated by how they construct time in nursing, patients feel close to them, a feeling they describe as "being on the same wavelength." What makes the art of nursing a "special" experience, according to patients, is their belief that the nurse cares about them. One patient stated:

When I was delivering and I couldn't get comfortable, she availed herself to hold my foot for me. I mean, my foot! When I think of feet, I think, you know, blah, but she held my foot.

Creating Opportunities for Fullness of Being

Preparing for personal well-being, making responsible decisions, and guiding self-expression describe the ways in which the nurse and patient cocreate opportunities for the patient in nursing. Each way characterizes a mode of interaction that reveals the mutual participation inherent to the process of nursing. Mutual participation in these modes of interaction illustrates the nature of the nurse's help in the art of nursing.

Preparation for life transitions occurs through informing patients and discussing feelings and options. The nurse and patient engage in a reciprocal process of sharing information. The nurse offers information necessary for the patient to make informed choices. The patient responds to this information by sharing personal information—desires, feelings, personal history, and hopes for the future. Participants state that this sharing helps discover the meaning a particular event has in a patient's life and assists with informed choice and planning. Mary commented on her experience of being informed by Gretchen:

> *They [Gretchen and her colleagues] automatically start with the teaching. They probe into your feelings and into your concerns. They answer all the questions they can. They give you pamphlets on things to eat. They educate you right off. They are concerned with your health. They want you to have the best experience you can.*

When nurses welcome patients' feelings, respect their wishes, and honor their need for self-expression, they help patients choose options that are in their best interest. By teaching, nurses inform patients about choices they can make. Knowing and understanding the patients' desires, hopes, and aims enables the nurses to honor the choices made and give the kind of caring that is responsible to the patient. By integrating knowledge inherent to nursing with knowledge of the unique person, the nurses cocreate and work toward an agreed-on aim in a manner that is consistent with the patients' desires.

Assisting patients to make choices describes the teaching nurses do in order to help in decision making. When nurses acknowledge patients' rights to choose and provide information necessary for informed choice, patients state that they feel supported by the nurses. According to the participants, the nurse and patient plan together the manner in which decisions will be carried out when both are informed. Decision making in the art of nursing involves assisting and acknowledging patients' decisions. By continuously inquiring, the nurse makes sure the patient is comfortable with the plan and understands the freedom to change a decision based on developing circumstances.

Coaching and following through constitute two ways nurses guide patients. The nurse provides safe passage for the patient by guiding the patient's self-expression through the plan. One patient responded to the nurse's coaching by giving feedback about the effectiveness as the experience unfolded:

> *She would make suggestions about how I could be comfortable while in that position. Sometimes no matter how much you are prepared beforehand you seem to forget it all at times. She would bring it back. She'd say, "How about trying to put your foot here" or "How about pressing this way or pushing that way." She had to remind me, like, four or five times. I know she was repeating it to me but I would forget because of the moment. The way she said it was very comforting, very nice.*

Participants state that frequent contact, checking up, and being thorough helps with following through and guides activities to complete a cycle of transition from being in the moment to realizing the fullness of the future.

A Transcendent Togetherness

In the art of nursing, a transcendent togetherness depicts the liberating experience of a emancipatory relationship that develops. By being faithful in the relationship of nursing with its practice, the nurse and patient cocreate an experience of nursing as liberating. Together, the patient and nurse feel closely synchronized in a union working effectively toward an identifiable and mutually agreed-on aim.

The intimate union of togetherness that bonds the nurse and patient into a *friendship* describes a relationship of nursing as a transcendent experience for the patient and nurse. Recognizing, feeling, and knowing that caring exists, the patient and nurse create a relationship beyond that of a working association. Patients describe feeling safe, secure, and bonded to the nurse. They trust that the nurse respects, safeguards, and enhances their wholeness of being by working with them—the hallmark of this intimate union. They know that, whatever happens, they can rely on the integrity of the nurse as a person and a professional, the practice of nursing, and the situation's evolving within the context of their decisions:

> *I had that feeling of being accepted, of being taken care of, of being loved, of being understood and being a part of it. It's like a big family there. You're part of a family and it transpires. It's more like you gain a friendship.*

The practice of nursing as a synchronized union of the patient and nurse working effectively toward a common aim constituted a feeling of mutual liberation and appreciation on the part of the patient and nurse. By enspiriting, supporting, and comforting, the nurse emancipates the patient; together they transcend the reality of the present and realize their potential for fullness of being. Enspiriting encompasses the togetherness of the patient and nurse as they create nursing as a "spiritual experience." Based in empathizing, intuiting, respecting, and trusting, a reciprocal spirituality occurs, for the nurse and patient, that entails knowing beyond the immediate reality.

The spirituality of this togetherness speaks of the quality of knowing that characterizes the support and depth of the nurse's help in the art of nursing:

> *You were like this little ghost. It was like you weren't really there. You were there but you weren't. I didn't feel like she was another person with other ideas, values, or goals. It was just like we were there together.*

The nurse knows how to encourage and reassure the patient by supporting the person's integrity (choice and control) and competence to care for oneself. This support originates from a holistic and humanistic perspective of a person and empowers patients to have faith in the decisions they make by maintaining control and feeling positive about themselves.

The feeling of comfort that transpires in the art of nursing is different from the notion of comfort as simply the absence of pain. Comfort describes the experience of soothing, easing, belonging, calming, and believing in what is transpiring. This comfort enables patients to transcend the moment. During times described as transcendence, being comfortable helped the patient to grow as a person.

The liberation that occurs with the nurse and patient reflects the personal transformation that transpires beyond the present moment. Patients describe feeling emancipated by the nurse's caregiving. Frequently, they express the belief that they have "grown as individuals and families." By entrusting, patients develop positive beliefs about their abilities and take responsibility for the experience of life transitions:

I feel like I became closer. I felt a lot more confident as far as knowing that I was okay. I felt very different after delivering this baby, after having this experience, because I felt that I'm on the same wavelength. When you're together with someone on the same wavelength, you're not constantly being banged up against the wall. You feel like you're doing fine and everything's great. We're all going to work together and your decisions that you make are always great. You feel so confident you can make the right decisions. You feel so confident when you're finished. You feel like when you care so much you enable yourself. You [the nurse] led me to make decisions, educated me, led me by your experiences that I just felt much more whole. It was just very joyous, very fulfilling to feel as one family, to feel that you're doing the right thing, that this is normal and you're intelligent enough to make the right decisions and they're going to help you. I think the biggest thing in having a child here with Marilyn [the nurse] was our family changed more so because it was more of a family experience. It wasn't just me and the baby. It was more of a family growth. You were a lot different. We felt a lot more comfortable. It seems like the family bond was more cemented together. We were glued together more because everyone's concerns were dealt with here.

Patients comment that the nurse's caring freed them and gave them an opportunity to become confident and self-reliant. Nurses describe feeling joy that they "make a difference" in the quality of life for patients. Feeling peaceful about the help that is given characterizes the art of nursing from other practices. Nurses and patients appreciate one another and the cocreated experience. The art of nursing as an extraordinary way of being together emerged as a transcendent togetherness; a depth of relating, a comprehensiveness of practicing, and a creation of opportunities also describe the context. A context of caring, the last metatheme, characterizes the distinctiveness of the setting and conditions in which a transcendent togetherness emerges.

A Context of Caring

Nursing exists as an extension of the philosophy of nursing into the context, a supportive setting sustaining the practice of nursing as art. By instituting values that express nursing as an art, the nursing philosophy enfolds into the setting and creates a safe, receptive environment for patients who identify their needs for help and make decisions with the nurse about their care. A nurse conveyed this view:

The philosophy here is basic to letting the patients be who they are, what they are, who they want to be, giving them more responsibility. I think the whole philosophy is really different from the [hospital]. Hospitals are trying to change, but there's still an element there that needs to control each person, tell the patient what to do, when to do it.

Values that underpin nursing, as described in the first four metathemes, include: honoring a person's integrity, understanding the interconnectedness of life and wholeness of human being, committing to liberating people as the way to personal transformation, and developing a community that appreciates nursing as art. These values reflect a universal nature of art (Rader, 1979) and demonstrate how nurses *originate* nursing, *create* it as art, and *evolve* a context of caring.

Nursing, the primary source of caring and core service, characterizes the setting. Contextually described, it is an "atmosphere of caring." This distinct environment or center of nursing is a place where nurses have day-to-day authority for all decisions concerning the practice of nursing. The organization and practice exist distinctively for the purpose of providing nursing as the way of helping patients. Opportunities for creating nursing thrive in a culture of nursing solely accountable for practice:

A lot of the people at the Center are like that [referring to kindness, consideration, and concern]. Most of them that I dealt with are like that. When you walk into the Center, it's such a different atmosphere. The atmosphere is, like, when you walk into the building you know you are going to have that care and that atmosphere. It's just a caring atmosphere, that caring. You walk in the door and it's like walking into your Mom's house and everybody's home. It's really nice to know that you're cared for that way, that there's a special feeling for you and for your family, and your whole experience. It makes your experience so much more special. Just the whole experience, the way the people treated you and really helped us through it and were there for us.

The extension of caring beyond the interpersonal domain into the context of the organization and environment where nursing transpires constructs a comprehensive and coherent experience that gives the context of helping patients "a personality of its own." For nurses who practice the art of nursing, caring permeates beyond the human-to-human intersubjective moment and exists contextually as well. Time, place, and space reflect nurses originating nursing as art. For example, these nurses are expected and supported to take time to come to know patients; to be flexible in making choices, depending on individual preference and need; to cocreate nursing; and to innovatively meet the challenges presented during the process of nursing. In addition, the environment is deliberately designed to be aesthetically pleasing and offers "a safe haven," "a home away from home" for patients.

The Meaning of the Art of Nursing

The unity of meaning, *"a transcendence together in love—the true spirit of understanding caring that creates a liberating way of helping,"* emerged from the themes and metathemes explicating the essence of the art of nursing (Appleton, 1991, p. 88). Derived from the narrative descriptions, this meaning gives visibility to nursing as art and to the nurse who originates nursing by understanding it in relationship to the meaning of the patient's experience. The nurse as artist is concerned with coming to know the patient. By being focused on developing this knowledge from the perspective of a patient who is vulnerable and has needs, the nurse designs nursing—an intimately private experience. During an interview, a nurse told this story, which illustrates the nurse's knowledge of the meaning of a patient's experience:

> *There was a lady in the hospital who was going to have a stillborn baby. She knew about it ahead of time. So during labor I gave her physical and emotional support all through that. This was not a full-term baby. I think the gestation was only about 5 or 6 months. So the baby wasn't even fully formed. I talked to the parents and they wanted to see the baby. So we wrapped it up as nicely as we could and gave the baby to the parents. To see them and how happy they were even in their grief to be able to hold this baby. They were just amazed by its little hands and feet. They looked at the whole baby and they were marvelling over different things. Then, when they were ready, we took the baby down to the morgue, and it was like that was everything because you knew that everything had been taken care of then. They felt peaceful because they had a fulfillment of the whole experience.*

By coming to know patients' meanings of their life experiences, nurses design a way of helping patients that maintains their integrity, demonstrates an understanding of their vulnerability, and develops opportunities for patients to meet their desired outcome. When the nurse comes to know patients from a perspective that exceeds traditional science and models of health care, opportunities for nursing arise and both nurse and patient give of themselves freely, willingly, and lovingly to achieve a mutual aim. Their purpose ensues in a togetherness, a way of knowing and being with each other that transcends conventional human boundaries. This intimacy of the relationship in nursing is the foundation for synchronizing being/knowing/doing in a togetherness that develops nursing as an art—a liberating emancipation, as described by this nurse:

> *I think there is a balance of giving somebody something and getting something back. When I give myself, I think the art is, I get so much back. I don't even know what it is, but it's a sensation of being high that I get from a birth. I just get so high from it. I get so much back in return. I work hard at it, and again imparting [knowledge], trying to let that person see that they're the one [in control]. Empowering [people] so that they see that they're the ones creating what's going on.*

The metaphor of "the gift of self" portrays the art of nursing as it originates with the nurse and patient, and describes the giving and receiving of the nurse and patient (Appleton, 1991, p. 88). The unfolding creation of nursing as art lies in the gift of self. *In caring*, the nurse originates nursing by giving what it takes, and with the patient cocreates a unique way of helping that makes a difference in the patient's life. When nurses give of themselves as described in this research, the artificial boundaries between theory and life dissolve.

Schon (1984) suggested that reflective practice requires the effective use of specialized knowledge, which depends on the ability to restructure situations that are complex and uncertain. This ability is grounded in the practitioner's skill to frame the context in which to attend. The nurse's experience not only frames activity, but becomes an activity of originating, creating, and designing. Representing a skillful practice, the nurse synthesizes the inner act of knowing with the outer expression of faithful presence. In doing so, reflection enables the nurse to use both divergent and convergent thinking, thereby creating skillful doing. Simply stated, nurses act on what they know in their experience with patients and will abandon technique or theory if it is not helpful with achieving the aims of patients. This is the nurse's gift of self, the commitment and ability to change existing experiences into preferred ones.

Helping, as distinguished in the art of nursing, "makes a difference" in the lives of patients. These nurses embody multiple ways of knowing; they come to know, create, and design nursing in the moment with each patient encountered. In so doing, they recognize and criticize their tacit understandings learned in repetitive experiences of nursing; they make new sense of uncertain and unique experience with each patient.

Originating nursing gives it form as art and exemplifies the skillfulness of the nurse by making what some of us do into a visible pattern of practice in which we display our nursing skills. As an emancipatory way of helping, the art of nursing offers a meaning of caring as liberating (Appleton, 1991).

IMPLICATIONS OF A PARADIGM OF ORIGINATING NURSING

Specific implications of this paradigm emphasize the intersubjective and contextual nature of the art of nursing. The intersubjective essence of art reveals the importance of the patient as the core concern of the nurse and describes the way being there develops as knowledge of caring. The significance of the patient's integrity to the experience of well-being and desired outcomes gives new meaning to the nurse's helping.

Empathizing, intuiting, respecting, and trusting occur in activities of preparing, deciding, and guiding that form a process of helping described as being-with each other in understanding.

When the nurse is there for and with patients, meaningful relating and creating transpire to form a friendship. What is important about the nurse as a friend is the mutually confirming experience of coming to know, acknowledge, and respect each other. Ultimately, harmony is cocreated and exemplifies the nurse's skillfulness in helping in caring.

A transcendent togetherness illustrates this further when the nurse and patient intimately bond to create an enspiriting, supporting, and comforting way to transcend the immediate moment. The nurse and patient achieve a potential for fullness of being and portray the intersubjective nature of the relationship in the art of nursing as emancipatory and liberating.

A transcendent togetherness exemplifies nursing at its finest and perhaps suggests that knowledge of nursing is also spiritual in that it is freeing. A transcendent togetherness holds profound implications for the profession. Specifically, such togetherness recognizes that the art of nursing is a liberating way of helping patients who then are the source of ongoing action, as exemplified in this participant's remarks:

> I felt very important and I felt more intrigued to take care of things. If it were my diet, she said, "Oh, you gained a little bit of weight this month. What did you do?" Oh, well, I did this. "Well, you don't need to eat that." Just taking that little bit of concern made me feel more like, "Oh God, I do need to do better and I don't need to eat this or do that." It made me feel better about myself. It gave me more self-confidence and [I was] ready to take care of things and follow through on what she said.

This perspective deepens the significance of the profession to make an emancipatory difference in health care.

The art of nursing gives caring a meaning of liberating help. Grounding caring in a paradigm of nursing as art takes the experience of nursing beyond the notion of aesthetic practice and offers a prototype of nursing as art comprising an ontology, epistemology, axiology, and praxis gestalt. The nature of science in nursing is reconciled by the nurse as artist. In originating nursing, the nurse weaves the diverse sources of knowledge—basic, applied, and practical—with the unknown into a quality of caring experienced as liberating help (Appleton, 1993). The artificial boundaries between sources of knowledge disappear and a unified, novel experience occurs. Ultimately, a new paradigm of art in which to understand nursing practice is constructed.

REFERENCES

Appleton, C. (1991). The gift of self: The meaning of the art of nursing. *Dissertation Abstracts International, 52,* 12B. (University Microfilms No. 92-15, 314).

Appleton, C. (1993). The art of nursing: The experience of patients and nurses. *Journal of Advanced Nursing, 18*(6), 892–899.

Glasser, B., & Strauss, A. (1967). *The discovery of grounded theory: Strategies for qualitative research.* New York: Aldine.

Husserl, E. (1970). *The crisis of European sciences and transcendental phenomenology: An introduction to phenomenological philosophy.* (D. Carr, Trans.). Evanston, IL: Northwestern University Press.

Nightingale, F. (1969). *Notes on nursing: What it is, and what it is not.* New York: Dover.

Nutting, A., & Dock, L. (1912). *A history of nursing: The evolution of nursing systems from earliest times to the foundations of the first English and American training schools for nurses* (Vols. I–IV). New York: Putnam.

Rader, M. (Ed.). (1979). *A modern book of esthetics: An anthology.* New York: Holt, Rinehart and Winston.

Ray, M. (1990). Phenomenological method for nursing research. In N. Chaska (Ed.), *The nursing profession: Turning points* (pp. 173–178). New York: McGraw-Hill.

Ray, M. (1991). Caring inquiry: The aesthetic process in the way of compassion. In D. A. Gaut & M. M. Leininger (Eds.), *Caring: The compassionate healer* (pp. 123–133). New York: National League for Nursing.

Reeder, F. (1987). The phenomenological movement. *Image: The Journal of Nursing Scholarship, 19*(3), 150–152.

Reeder, F. (1988). Hermeneutics. In B. Sarter (Ed.), *Paths to knowledge* (pp. 193–238). New York: National League for Nursing.

Schon, D. A. (1984). *The reflective practitioner: How professionals think in action.* New York: Basic Books.

Stewart, I. (1929). The science and art of nursing (Editorial). *Nursing Education Bulletin, 2,* 1.

van Manen, M. (1984). Practicing phenomenological writing. *Phenomenology + Pedagogy, 5*(3), 230–241.

van Manen, M. (1990). *Researching lived experience: Human science for an action-sensitive pedagogy.* New York: SUNY Press.

Part II

Art as Learning

6

Integrating the Arts and Humanities into Nursing Education

Elizabeth R. Bruderle
Theresa M. Valiga

THE HUMANITIES IN NURSING EDUCATION

Nursing is an art; and if it is to be made an art,
it requires an exclusive devotion, as hard a preparation,
*   as any painter's or sculptor's work;*
for what is the having to do with dead canvas or cold
*   marble,*

The authors wish to acknowledge the contributions of Phoebe Kennel Haupert, MSN, RN, to portions of this manuscript. They also wish to acknowledge the graduate students who, over the years, have enrolled in the elective course, "Creative Teaching Strategies in Nursing: Using the Humanities," and contributed their ideas, suggestions, and enthusiasm about the humanities and nursing.

117

compared with having to do with the living body—the
temple of God's spirit?
It is one of the Fine Arts;
I had almost said, the finest of the Fine Arts.

Florence Nightingale

There is no question that the practice of nursing is challenging and ever-changing and that it takes place in a health care delivery system that is complex, relies on experts in a number of fields, and is, in and of itself, ever-changing. In order to practice professional nursing in this environment, nurses and nurse educators must have not only a sound scientific foundation but also a concern for and commitment to humanistic health care, which Donaldson (1983) maintained is the uniqueness of nursing.

A humanistic perspective involves caring, but it also encompasses a broader awareness and understanding of people's concerns and feelings, the contexts in which they live, their cultures, and the ways they live in the world. Nurses interact with people at critical junctures in their lives, at times when humanistic care is most needed. To provide humanistic care, practitioners must have self-knowledge, an understanding of the separateness and individuality of others, and an ability to integrate and connect the experiences of others within themselves (Wilson, 1974). Because the humanities address the responses of human beings to a variety of experiences, they offer nurse educators a unique strategy to facilitate the integration of the science of nursing with its critical complement, the art of nursing.

In a study of 91 senior baccalaureate students and alumnae, Peck and Jennings (1989) found that although the students and alumnae generally thought that the liberal arts and humanities were an important aspect of their educational experience, they believed that they themselves—not their nursing faculty—made the links between liberal arts and nursing. We might be encouraged by the finding that students (and alumnae even more so) valued the liberal arts in their preparation as nurses, but the authors of the study apparently defined liberal arts as including biology, chemistry, English, nutrition, psychology, and sociology (p. 410), and *not* in terms of philosophy, literature, religion, history, and the fine arts, as they typically are defined in the literature. Thus, we must be cautious in our enthusiasm. In addition, the finding that faculty were not particularly influential in helping students "make the links" leads one to question whether faculty truly value the liberal arts or see the "links" themselves.

The legitimate concern that nursing faculty should attend to the integration of nursing with the arts and humanities was expressed almost a quarter of a century ago by Dickoff and James (1970) and by Priest (1970). These authors, noting that we are educating nurses for their profession *and* as human beings living in a world of living people, acknowledged the importance of the humanities in that process.

Boyer (1987), who suggested integrating the liberal arts *into* professional education, argued that the greatest advantages from such integration will be realized when it touches on the *major* and is not limited to the early years of the curriculum or the general education component.

Students need to learn to *blend* liberal arts and professional values and abilities, and the two need to "depend on each other" (Armour & Fuhrmann, 1989, p. 2). Indeed, as Curtis (1985, p. 10) noted, we need to address and resolve the "ancient dichotomy that has plagued American higher education at least since the founding of the land grant colleges," namely, the "split" between liberal and professional education.

Thus, this is not a new concern for educators in general or for nurse educators in particular; however, it is not clear whether the blending of the humanities with nursing has been achieved adequately. We would do well to heed Newell's (1989) suggestion: Don't just "'[parcel] out' chunks of the curriculum" (p. 69) to the liberal arts, but explore other approaches to blending the liberal arts and nursing, including "a greater use of humanities, arts, and social science content *in nursing courses*" (p. 69) [emphasis added].

Lee (1986, p. 62) asserted that "the art and craft of teaching requires that one has a repertoire of teaching moves and is skilled in their use, but more important, that one is able to draw on educational imagination and invent new moves that advance the students from one place to another along the intellectual path." The integration of the arts and humanities into nursing courses is a "new move" for most nurse educators and one that may be uncomfortable. In this chapter, we ask nurse educators to consider the outcomes of using the humanities, as described herein, and to be open to their relationship to characterizations of critical thinking, their relevance to nursing practice, and the possibilities that await.

WHY THE HUMANITIES

The "humanities" may be thought of as the branch of knowledge that deals with what it means to be human, to live authentically, and to share with others. The humanities focus on people: what they experience, how they respond to and interpret the world around them, and what meaning they make of it all. The humanities provide for a liberal education and incorporate the disciplines of philosophy, literature, history, religion, the fine arts, and other arts. But as Newell (1989) pointed out, liberal education "is not the exclusive province of any set of academic departments or administrative divisions" (p. 69).

Helping individuals learn what it means to be human involves facilitating their examination of their attitudes toward life, the place of the individual in society, the nature of our common humanity, the significance of human endeavors, and the relationships and responsibilities of individuals to one another. The humanities allow and encourage unique interpretations of events and situations, acknowledge the importance of feelings in our lives, focus on people and what they experience, provide opportunities for individuals to confront and deal with uncertainty, and promote individuality. They are, indeed, humanistic.

Many students think of the humanities merely as courses that must be endured in order to earn a baccalaureate degree. Many individuals also view the arts and humanities, as Bartol (1986, p. 21) noted, as "a fine veneer that enables [us] to communicate socially with others and provides an interesting diversion to manage stress" (p. 21). The arts and humanities often are seen as providing little more than bits and pieces of trivial knowledge that may be useful at cocktail parties or in *Jeopardy!* or a similar game. The humanities are much more. The following list suggests, in no order of rank, their primary goals and ancillary benefits:

- Help us avoid routine;
- Introduce mysteries and unknowns;
- Develop deep and lasting personal values;
- Heighten our sense of choice and decision;
- Stretch our imaginations;
- "[P]rovide contexts for the decisions we must make as a people by raising questions of social purpose" (Text of Cheney's Report . . . , 1988, p. A17);
- Provide images of human reality and possibility;
- Provide a historical context and connections with and insights to the past;
- "[E]nlarge [our] understanding by showing us we are not the first generation to grapple with moral dilemmas" (Text of Cheney's Report . . . , 1988, p. A17);
- Awaken or elucidate our beliefs and values and help us clarify the personal values that guide our actions;
- Expose or sensitize us to certain realities;
- "[C]onvey how the ideas and ideals of our civilization have evolved, thus providing a basis for understanding other cultures" (Text of Cheney's Report . . . , 1988, p. A18);
- Increase our social consciousness;
- Help us understand time, process, and change;
- "[P]rovide a framework for lifelong learning about ourselves and the world in which we live" (Text of Cheney's Report . . . , 1988, p. A18);
- Help us grasp the state of the world in which we live and act;
- Expose us to new ideas, perspectives, and areas of knowledge;
- "[F]ree the mind from ignorance, prejudice, and slavish dependence on other minds" (Newell, 1989, p. 69);

- Increase our sensitivity and our sense of compassion and empathy;
- Accentuate the multifaceted nature of the world;
- Develop new insights into problem solving, decision making, and resolution of personal conflicts;
- Help us know ourselves and the world around us in very different ways;
- Liberate our potentials;
- Provide opportunities for private moments and reflection;
- Promote differences of opinion and points of view and support an acceptance of such differences;
- Inspire us;
- Encourage the expression of original ideas and personal perspectives;
- Promote intellectual, cultural, and personal growth, thereby developing the whole person;
- Call on and develop right-brain skills, thereby stimulating our creativity;
- Acknowledge the legitimacy of intuitive thinking;
- Promote synthesis rather than reductionism;
- Help us appreciate and manage the diversity, ambiguity, and uncertainty that characterize our world;
- Heighten our perceptions and feelings;
- Foster the development of an inquiring mind;
- Help develop greater insights;
- "[H]elp people understand themselves in historical, cultural and aesthetic terms" (Arts, Education and Americans Panel, cited in Lee, 1986, p. 62);
- Provide us with broader choices and more options;
- Provide alternate ways to introduce and reinforce learning;
- Initiate us into the artistic, aesthetic domain without trying to make artists or poets out of us;
- Spotlight the shared values of knowledge that bind people together as a society;

- Promote interdisciplinary perspectives and the relationship of one discipline to another;
- "[W]aken us from the numbness that all too frequently accompanies routine" (Bartol, 1986, p. 23).

If nurse educators are to attempt the integration of the arts and humanities *with nursing* and *in nursing courses and learning experiences,* some guideposts are needed. Specifically, one needs to consider how to find or uncover appropriate works of art and what criteria to consider in selecting and using them.

CRITERIA FOR THE SELECTION AND USE OF THE ARTS AND HUMANITIES

As when they are using any other teaching/learning strategy, nurse educators must be guided by some criteria when considering the use of the arts and humanities to facilitate student learning of nursing concepts. Those criteria are varied. General criteria are discussed here; some are discussed in greater detail in relation to specific art forms.

First, one must consider the philosophy and mission of the university and the nursing program and how well the art form "fits" with them. A second criterion to guide one's selection of a work of art is its availability and accessibility. Third, one should consider the amount of time it will take students to actually use the particular art form within or outside the classroom. In addition to these criteria, nurse educators must consider the students' (and their colleagues'!) attitudes toward such creative approaches to learning, as well as their own comfort with the subject matter at hand and the approach being used. Finally, nurse educators need to consider cost, the relevance of the work of art to the learning objectives, the developmental level and nursing knowledge base (i.e., the "sophistication") of the students involved, and the timeliness of the material.

Given the relevance of the arts and humanities to nursing education and the criteria one needs to consider prior to selecting and using such approaches, let us now examine some specific art forms. In each instance, the art form will be described, the advantages and disadvantages of using the art form will be summarized, resources for locating such art forms will be suggested, and several specific examples of how the art form can be used in nursing education will be offered. These discussions are not intended to be all-inclusive or complete; rather, they introduce the variety of ways in which nurse educators can attend to the integration of the arts and humanities into nursing education.

LITERATURE

Literature, a form of learning included among the humanities, provides insight into human nature through the written depiction of real or imagined experiences (Perrine, 1983). Through literary works, students can experience reality vicariously and can begin to develop the sensitivity to others that is so central to nursing. Novels, short stories, and children's books are discussed here as examples of relevant literary works.

Among the numerous resources available to help in identifying appropriate novels, short stories, and children's books are personal reading experiences, book reviews, and best-seller lists (e.g., in *The New York Times* or *The New Yorker*), anthologies, and bookstore browsing. In addition, casual conversation with friends, nursing colleagues, or faculty in other disciplines, such as librarians and English professors, often help in identifying books and stories that may have relevance.

There are several *advantages* to using literature as a teaching strategy. The vast number of works in existence provides an almost endless supply of assignment possibilities. Students can be exposed to good writing and encouraged to recognize the value of non-nursing material to their overall development. In addition, the solitary nature of reading tends to foster introspection and the development of self-awareness. Discussions based on assigned readings offer an alternative to the lecture format and thus facilitate active learning and class participation. During such interactions, critical thinking and problem-solving capabilities are enhanced as students consider the variety of interpretations offered by faculty and fellow students. Finally, the integration of nursing content with the human experiences described in the literature stimulates students' interest and increases retention of content (Germain, 1986).

The increased preparation time required of the faculty members is one of the *disadvantages* to the use of literature. Although it is not necessary for professors to be literary critics, they must read the proposed assignment critically to ascertain appropriateness and factual accuracy of any scientific content. In addition, the need for study guides, relevant questions to guide reading, and adequate class time for debriefing and evaluation must be considered. Practical concerns related to the availability of a large number of copies of assigned books and the cost of some books also must be addressed as possible disadvantages.

Novels

Novels are fictional, prose narratives in which a plot unfolds through the actions, thoughts, and speech of the characters. The purposes of novels are to entertain, instruct, and inform, and these aims are accomplished through the fictionalization of human themes, the very issues that nurses encounter on a daily basis. Novels are generally longer and often span a more extended period of time than other literary forms. In addition, novels may include a variety of settings, in-depth character studies, and lengthy descriptions.

The length of many novels, an obvious disadvantage to their use, can be addressed by assigning carefully selected and well-explained portions of a book. Or, in an ideal educational setting, the same novel could be assigned by more than one professor to meet a variety of course objectives. For example, *The Great Santini* (Conroy, 1976) could be assigned by an English professor for a literary critique and by a Nursing professor to present the concepts of family dynamics and interpersonal communication.

Novels enable educators to address a variety of behavioral objectives ranging from simple identification to complex levels of analysis and synthesis, to introduce and expand on specific concepts, and to evaluate learning. Richard Adams' (1972) *Watership Down* is an excellent example of a novel with broad applicability. This beautifully written book describes power structures, community dynamics, and the relation between leaders and followers through the vehicle of four rabbit warrens (Futrell, 1983). The rabbit warrens, each depicting a different leadership style, serve as highly descriptive complements to the didactic material typically presented in textbooks. For the beginning student, this book could serve as an introduction to the concept of leadership and an examination of leadership theories; at a more advanced level, students learning to formulate leadership strategies could be assigned to propose an alternative to Bigwig's authoritarian style or to lead a discussion of the advantages and disadvantages of life in Hazel's participative community.

Short Stories

Brevity is the characteristic that primarily distinguishes the short story from the novel. Angus (1962) suggested that the "strict limits" (p. 7) of the short story challenge authors to a high level of creativity rarely achieved by those who write novels. This unique quality is a distinct advantage to nurse educators seeking appropriate literary works to address the learning objectives of their students.

Young-Mason (1991) has recommended Conrad's short story, *The Secret Sharer,* to sensitize nursing students to the nuances of the nurse–patient relationship and to the concept of professionalism. Conrad's description of a novice sea captain's first command provides students with a realistic experience analogous to their own initial professional experiences. Through this literary work, students can identify with the young captain as he makes decisions, considers consequences, and accepts responsibility for his actions. As students share their perceptions of the character's values and judgments, they gain insight based on an imaginary, nonthreatening experience. Younger (1990) referred to this phenomenon as "the experience of life without its costs" (p. 42).

Children's Stories

Today's readers of children's books enjoy a wide selection and a broad range of types within the genre. Among the possibilities, one finds traditional fairy tales, ageless classics, and contemporary literature (Goldreich, 1977). Traditional works, although ever popular and not without considerable value, are essentially fantasies, complete with happy endings. The more current offerings for children appear to reflect modern psychology: they approach life experiences from a realistic and rational perspective. Approach notwithstanding, Cardozo (1992) suggested that simple stories that recognize those emotions that are distinctly human remain among the best. Younger (1990) found that the significant insights evident in such stories are perceived by readers of all ages, "though with different levels of meaning" (p. 42). Children are repeatedly drawn to certain stories without a clear understanding of their attraction; adults, however, find messages in the simplicity of children's books that enhance their understanding of complex issues.

The concepts of death and dying are typical of complex issues that can be introduced to nursing students through the reading and discussing of children's books. *A Taste of Blackberries* (Smith, 1973) is a child's first-person account of his attempts to confront the meaning of death after his best friend dies of a bee sting. Through the "aesthetic distance" (Bartol, 1986, p. 23) of the young boy's words, the reader participates in the child's experience and gains some understanding of the nature of human responses to the mystery of death.

MacLachlan's (1992) brief but articulately written *Journey* describes, again in the first person, an 11-year-old boy's search for a personal history after he is abandoned by his mother. The book also addresses the ways in which different generations confront loss. As students share the narrator's thoughts, they are able to reflect on their own experiences with loss or to explore loss vicariously. This turning inward for meaning is the foundation for compassion, a quality that may well describe the essence of nursing (Younger, 1990).

TELEVISION AND FILMS

Although not considered as among the humanities, per se, television and films are discussed here because they are the media through which literary works are often presented to the public. Because the advantages and disadvantages of using both forms are similar, they are discussed together. Differences unique to each are addressed separately.

The most significant *advantage* to the use of television and films is their enormous popularity. Viewers of all ages relate to both as forms of entertainment, communicators of information, and transmitters of knowledge. In addition, the current generation of students is well-oriented to the use of television as a teaching strategy.

Within a controlled time period, students obtain a global perspective of a given experience or relationship without the need to exert much in the way of energy or imagination. However, the dual stimuli of sight and sound create the potential for a powerful and long-lasting impact on students.

One distinct *disadvantage* of using either form as a teaching strategy is society's perception of their purpose as purely entertainment. To avoid questions about academic value, then, it is incumbent on faculty to ascertain that students understand the objectives of an assignment that requires viewing television or a film. In addition, faculty need to be aware of the tremendous influence that both media have on the formation of attitudes and values and of the potential for stereotyping related to racial and ethnic groups, male–female relationships, and developmental levels.

Among the practical issues that should be considered when using television and film are the need to preview the work for quality and applicability, the time required for students to view a film or program, and the cost of renting films, videotapes, and hardware for classroom use. The need to schedule follow-up discussion within a reasonable period of time is critical to facilitate learning.

Resources for identifying television programs and films include anthologies (many of which are annotated and categorized according to subject matter), entertainment reviews in newspapers and on television (e.g., *Siskel and Ebert*), and contact with specific groups that support programming, such as The Center for Creative Leadership. One's personal viewing and experiences or those of others are often the most fruitful sources of information on relevant shows or films.

Television

Television is a tremendously powerful and pervasive medium that exerts considerable influence on all facets of modern experience. The messages that it projects are influenced not only by societal trends but also by the need to attract audiences. Complex issues often are portrayed as simple and easily resolved within a half-hour time frame. For this reason, educators need to assess carefully the programs that are assigned for educational purposes. Nonetheless, there is an almost inexhaustible supply of high-quality, easily accessible viewing options.

The myriad "talk shows" available provide a vehicle for introduction to and observation and evaluation of the communication process. Students assigned to watch Phil Donahue could compare and contrast their findings with those of a group who observed Oprah Winfrey. A study guide could assist students to focus on specific factors such as the setting, the effectiveness of the communication strategies, the interviewer's nonverbal messages, and the verbal and nonverbal responses of the interviewees. The assignment of two or more programs to specific groups would allow students to increase their experience without an additional input of time and would foster group sharing and communication/reporting skills.

Situation comedies such as *The Bill Cosby Show* and *Cheers,* which can be found in rerun programming, are useful for gaining insight into interpersonal relationships, human behavior, and problem solving. A care plan based on the psychosocial needs of "Sam Malone," or goal statements and nursing interventions designed to address ineffective family coping among "the Huxtables" can be implemented in a safe and nonthreatening manner. Students can practice problem-solving skills by writing alternative endings for an assigned episode, using theories presented in class.

In addition to careful use of commercial television, faculty will find a variety of resources among the documentaries and educationally oriented offerings of public television. *To Live Until You Die* and *The Miracle of Life* are representative of programming that is available (Matza, 1988).

Films

Commercially prepared, full-length films have been a mainstay of the mass media for almost a century. From the earliest black-and-white offerings of the silent-film era to today's marvels of sight, sound, and color, films have provided society with extraordinarily rich and diverse experiences. Individuals have screamed with Bette Davis, cried with Debra Winger, and imagined themselves buried alive with Harrison Ford. With the advent of videocassette recorders, disadvantages such as film length, ticket cost for movie theater attendance, and availability have been eliminated. Students can now view films privately, repeat segments of the films if they wish, and reflect on all or selected scenes at their own pace.

Woody Allen's *Hannah and Her Sisters* (1986) is a complex study of family relationships, alcoholism, death, and love. Despite the serious nature of the issues addressed, Allen directed the film from a humorous perspective. The result is that the viewer is afforded insight into some of life's most profound experiences while being entertained. This film lends itself well to the viewing selected vignettes and offers significant content for discussion. *A Raisin in the Sun* (Petrie, 1961) explores some of the same concepts from the perspective of an African American family.

Poetry

Poems are like dreams: in them you put what you don't know you know.

Adrienne Rich

Poetry, one of the earliest art forms, is thought to have magical value in many societies. In many cultures, it is believed that understanding the power of the lyrics and rhythm inherent in poetry enables one to comprehend the laws of nature and the universe (*The Volume* Library, 1982). It also is believed that poetry allows one to delve into human experiences, thus capturing the nature of being.

Poems express feelings and thoughts in an imaginative way, using emotional, rhythmic language. In the teaching of nursing, they can be used to set a mood when introducing new material, convey a point of view, open discussion on a particular topic, or ascertain students' feelings and perceptions.

In addition to this *advantage* of wide applicability, poetry is practical to use, allows for individual expression and interpretation in the absence of any "rights or wrongs," is familiar to students, and can be used inside or outside the classroom with ease and minimal time. The *disadvantages* of using poetry to teach nursing stem from a hesitation to be so expressive, to seek the possible meanings behind the emotional expressions of others, or to deal with the emotion that may be evoked by the reading of a moving poem.

One might also assert that the inability to find appropriate poems is a disadvantage, but this claim is unjustified. Literally thousands of poems are available in library books, and they often are classified by topic (e.g., loss, birth, power). In addition to these generic sources, poems often are published in nursing journals (e.g., *The American Journal of Nursing, Perspectives in Psychiatric Care*) or in books specific to health care issues (Coles, 1978; Mukand, 1988). Finally, nurses themselves express their many significant experiences through poetry (Krysl, 1988, 1989; Oiler, 1983), and these can be a rich source for use in teaching.

Among the more familiar poets whose work can be used in nursing education are Dylan Thomas, Edgar Allen Poe, Robert Frost, Alfred Lord Tennyson, Khalil Gibran, and Rudyard Kipling. Thomas's "Do Not Go Gentle into that Good Night" is a plea not to merely accept one's life and death but to fight, to strive, to struggle, and to work toward goals; it can be used to initiate a discussion about aging, death, or the ethical dilemmas associated with life support systems. "Annabel Lee," by Poe, conveys the love, loss, and anger experienced by a man upon the death of his beloved wife, and it may be useful in helping students understand the bonds between individuals and how they grow over the years.

The concepts of human interaction and differing perspectives are addressed in Frost's "Meeting and Passing," a poem about two people coming from different directions, meeting, talking, and moving on. His "The Road Not Taken" can be used to discuss the concepts of choice and decision making. Tennyson's "I Wait" addresses the pain and hopefulness of waiting and how the sweetness of anticipation can be overshadowed by the fear of the unknown—situations inevitably encountered by the clients for whom nursing students care.

In *The Prophet*, Gibran (1973) offers words of wisdom about many of life's situations, including working, giving to others, experiencing joy and sorrow, and dealing with children, all of which are relevant to nurses. Kipling's "If" challenges us to think about leadership, strength, and change—concepts that have meaning for nursing practice.

Finally, students can be invited to write their own poems as a way to express their feelings and insights. This can be done through free-flowing poems, imitating Peck's (1993) use of poem-writing in helping students learn about mobility and activity in the elderly. A more structured approach is haiku, a 700-year-old art form of 17 syllables expressed in three lines containing 5, 7, and 5 syllables respectively. Haikus are simple to compose and easily learned. They "(1) provide a creative form of verbal expression; (2) increase sensitivity to selected topics and issues; (3) provide the reader with a chance to share the mood of the writer; and (4) evaluate or summarize thoughts and feelings about a particular class or learning experience" (Gustafson, 1979, p. 59). Thus, the writing of poetry by students themselves can be as valuable in nursing education as the reading of others' poetry.

THE FINE ARTS

The category of "fine arts" includes a variety of forms of artistic expression. The fine arts discussed here are paintings, sculpture, music, and photography, chosen for their relevance for nursing education. These teaching tools can be easily found in bookstores, libraries, local museums, college art departments, personal photo albums, and one's own community (e.g., the many public sculptural exhibits in New York, Boston, Philadelphia, and San Francisco). Donahue's (1988) book, *Nursing: The Finest Art,* will introduce readers to many relevant works of art.

Paintings

"A few drops of paint, deposited on a flat surface, can absorb the eye's sweetest moments" (Schier, 1988, p. 13). This statement captures the essence of paintings. If we have ideas to express, the proper medium is language, but if we have feelings to convey, the visual arts may be more powerful, and paintings are a most effective form of visual communication.

"All artists have the same intention, the desire to please; and art is most simply and most usually defined as an attempt to create pleasing forms" (Read, 1968, p. 18). Indeed, this representation of the visual world is the painter's expression of self and an attempt to arrange shape, color, texture, and content in a way that will elicit a pleasing reaction.

When examining art, the viewer must have "a perfectly open mind" (Read, 1968, p. 35) because the experience of viewing a painting is instantaneous. "[A]rt is not a code to be deciphered but an experience that awaits the sensitized eye" (Schier, 1988, p. 14). It provides for an almost liberating experience on the part of the viewer.

According to Read (1968, p. 266), "The function of art is not to transmit *feeling* so that others may experience the same *feeling.* . . . The real function of art is to express *feeling* and transmit *understanding.* " Thus, paintings have a great deal of value in nursing education.

Paintings, as a strategic medium for teaching nursing, have the *advantage* of presenting a pleasing stimulus to the learner and allowing each individual to express his or her own interpretation of the message conveyed through the work. Paintings can be extremely detailed, allowing for a thorough analysis of the situation depicted; or they can be quite simple, allowing for a clear, unencumbered presentation of an idea or emotion. In addition, paintings express every human emotion and every human situation, thereby establishing their relevance to many aspects of nursing education. Finally, numerous significant paintings are available from which to select.

There are, however, some *disadvantages* to using paintings; lack of accessibility and transportability are among the biggest deterrents. Museums may be miles from the university campus, and the university Art Department may have strict limitations on opening its collection to nonmajors. Even when a faculty member does find a painting that can be brought to the classroom, care must be taken in how it is transported and stored. Bookstores and art galleries often have excellent photographs or reasonably priced reproductions of famous paintings that can be purchased and transported quite easily—and perhaps used to decorate the faculty member's office in between class uses of the work!

There are many examples of paintings that convey concepts relevant to nursing. Grant Wood's "American Gothic," depicting a stoic, hard-working couple holding farming tools, represents the essence of stamina and discipline. An incredibly moving and graphic portrayal of suffering in the midst of squalor is David Alfaro Siqueiros' "Echo of a Scream"; this piece depicts the smallness and helplessness of a child in a confused world. Similar images of pain and suffering are evident in Edvard Monck's "The Cry" and "The Scream." Mary Cassatt's paintings portray human interactions, intimacy, and, in "The Bath," mother–infant bonding. Norman Rockwell's paintings represent many significant themes, including human needs (e.g., "The Four Freedoms") and common social and professional roles (e.g., "Before the Shot").

The discussion thus far has centered on having students view, study, respond to, and analyze paintings created by other individuals. There also may be great value in allowing students who have the interest and talent to paint pictures depicting relevant concepts as a way to express their understanding of those concepts. Students might be given the option of writing a formal term paper, writing a short story or a portfolio of poems, composing a song, or painting a picture to depict *their* personal conception of nursing's image or poverty or loss. Not only would such an exercise stimulate their creativity, but it would give them some degree of control over the course requirements they complete. The faculty member will find it much more exciting to evaluate the clarity of the meaning and understanding inherent in a variety of forms of expression than to read 20 or 30 very similar, traditional term papers.

Sculpture

What distinguishes sculpture as an art is its material and technique. Most other art forms involve the creation of a piece; sculpture can involve creating and building or cutting away. Michelangelo saw two types of sculpture: "the sort that is executed by cutting away from the block [of stone, marble, or wood] [and] the sort that is executed by building up" (Read, 1968, pp. 245-246).

Sculpture is a multidimensional art form that most approximates reality because it has length, width, and depth. Cellini thought that sculpture "is eight times as great as any other art . . . because a statue has eight views, and they must all be equally good" (Read, 1968, p. 244).

As is true with other art forms, sculpture can be used to express the appearance of things, express the reality of things, embody ideals, explore the unknown, or attempt to create a new order of reality. It, therefore, has the potential for being useful in nursing education.

The *advantages* to using sculpture in nursing education are that it *is* multidimensional, it can be touched and felt by students, and it is durable. Sculpture's *disadvantages* are that, like several other art forms discussed here, it may not be easily accessible or transportable, and faculty may not be aware of available works that might have relevance for selected educational experiences.

Among the pieces of sculpture that could be used in nursing education are Michelangelo's "Pieta," which conveys empathy, understanding, and compassion, and Rodin's "The Kiss," which communicates the concepts of intimacy and closeness. "The Standing Woman," by LaChaise, an enormous sculpture of a woman, depicts strength and power and could be used to facilitate a discussion of women and power. Nancy Fried's "Hanging Out," a sculpture of a woman's torso with one breast and one mastectomy scar, is an excellent stimulus for a discussion of cancer, loss, body image, or self-concept.

The idea of using sculpture and other art forms is not new to the nursing literature (Hoshiko, 1985; Loden, 1989). Several years ago, Hoshiko (1985) provided nursing faculty with a wonderful example of how sculpture and other art forms (particularly paintings) could be used to help students develop their diagnostic skills at a local art museum. The students were to wander throughout the museum and look at the various works of art, noting the nursing diagnosis(es) they would formulate about the conditions depicted in each piece. Particularly enjoyable was Hoshiko's description of the nursing diagnoses applicable to a knight in armor: "Anxiety, Alterations in Bowel Elimination (potential for constipation or incontinence), Alteration in Comfort (pain, itching), Impaired Verbal Communication, Deficit in Diversional Activity," and so on (Hoshiko, 1985, pp. 34-35). Imagine the fun the students had with this exercise, the lasting impression it made on them, and its effectiveness in helping them formulate nursing diagnoses. One wonders if these same outcomes could ever have been achieved through a lecture on the topic.

Music

Music is "the most abstract of all arts" (Wold & Cykler, 1967, p. 17). It provides a stimulus that allows the listener to interpret, in a personal way, the words, the sounds, and the feelings conveyed. There is no reality; there is merely the meaning given to the music by the listener.

Music "is inseparably connected with the social, economic, political, and religious pattern of its age" (Wold & Cykler, 1967, p. 4). Thus, it has the potential for helping listeners appreciate a culture's significant concerns, modes of expression, and progress (or lack thereof).

The music used in teaching nursing concepts can be classical or contemporary in nature, and students can listen to an entire work or one small passage. In addition, depending on the medium in which the work is available (record, cassette, compact disk), students can listen to it inside or outside the class.

The melody in a piece of music conveys emotions and feelings ranging from anger and hostility to sadness and depression or joy and happiness. This is done in abstract ways through the types of instruments selected, the predominantly high or low tones that comprise the work, the volume variations in the performance of the piece, and the intensity of the work. The addition of lyrics reduces this abstractness to some degree by providing actual verbal messages. Again, the particular words chosen, the emphases given to certain words or phrases, and the emotions conveyed through the human voice (e.g., sniffles, a cracking voice, a growl, a lilt), are integral to the message that is delivered.

The function of music, therefore, is not merely entertainment. Music encircles people and turns them from pure listeners to participants. Specific values are expressed and crystallized in music.

Aaron Copeland once said that the freely imaginative mind is the core of all vital music listening. Unfortunately, in the process of learning numerous "technical" skills, nursing students may develop into concrete thinkers, diminishing their creative and imaginative skills. One objective of using music in the teaching–learning process, therefore, is to allow the music to restore to the student's mind some of the emotional aspects of nursing's reality, which may be clouded by the demands of technology.

Music has numerous *advantages* in nursing education. It is an art form that most people like or at least can tolerate quite amiably. College-age students, in particular, have been reared in a music-oriented society, with music playing at home, in their dorms, in cars, in shopping malls, and in dentists' offices, and they are quite accustomed to the medium.

Music has the great advantage of being easily transportable. Using today's technology, it is easy to tape-record a musical piece and play it for a group of students. Using records or compact disks may be more difficult, but selections in these formats can be taped easily. There is a vast store of musical selections from which to choose. The nurse educator can easily find instrumental or vocal pieces to convey practically every conceivable concept.

What are the *disadvantages* of using music to teach nursing concepts? Perhaps one of the biggest disadvantages is attitudinal, on the part of faculty members themselves, their faculty colleagues, and students. Music may be thought of as frivolous—a "waste" of class time. Further, students may not appreciate the full significance of a piece of music. For example, students who were born in the 1970s may not understand the societal conditions of the 1960s that prompted songs about the destruction of the world, racial violence, and loss of innocence; if the faculty member does not provide the "backdrop" for this or other types of music, their significance may be lost to the students. If the words of a song are important to the learning objective, they must be made known to the students, and this may be difficult to accomplish. Finally, it often is necessary to listen to a piece of music several times before the ideas and emotions being conveyed can be appreciated. If music is to be played during class time and such time is limited, there may not be an opportunity for repetitions of the piece, and its full impact may be lost.

The concepts of loss, death, and mortality are conveyed through popular performers' renditions of contemporary songs like "Seasons in the Sun" (Terry Jacks) and "Dust in the Wind" (Kansas), as well as through classical pieces like the "Lamentation Symphony" composed by Haydn. James Taylor's recording of "You've Got a Friend" and The Brotherhood of Man's "United We Stand" address the ideas of caring, collaboration, and helping, as does "He Ain't Heavy, He's My Brother," sung by Neil Diamond. Helen Reddy's classic "I Am Woman" might stimulate a discussion of women's roles or women as leaders, "Ebony and Ivory" (Paul McCartney and Stevie Wonder) could prompt an exchange of ideas about cultural differences and collaboration; Harry Chapin's "Cat's in the Cradle" might be used to initiate or clarify material about intergenerational differences and communication. Finally, the many views and perspectives on change could be illustrated by comparing "Blowin' in the Wind" (Peter, Paul, and Mary), "Send in the Clowns" (Judy Collins), "The Times They Are a-Changin'" (Bob Dylan) and the Beatles' "Revolution."

Music is an enjoyable and extremely effective medium for the expression of thoughts and emotions. By having students listen to the music of their own and others' cultures, they can appreciate various conditions of the human existence. By creating their own music or lyrics, students can represent their personal ideas and feelings. For example, several years ago, a song entitled "If I Ruled the World" was recorded by Tony Bennett. If students in a nursing leadership course were asked to write their own words for this song or another such as "The Impossible Dream," an opportunity for aspiring and creative expression would be provided that might not be available through other teaching-learning approaches. In the assignment, students might learn something quite important about themselves, their values, and their leadership styles.

Photography

Photographs are of three kinds: (1) art photographs, (2) documentary photographs, and (3) personal photographs. All have potential relevance to nursing education.

A photograph is a representation of reality, achieved through the use of a camera. The camera "'takes' what is put in front of it [and] captures the subject without further judgment" (Beloff, 1985, p. 23). "In one sense a photograph promises reality and truth and scientific precision . . . in another it is the domain of art . . . [and] in yet another it holds magic and mystery" (Beloff, 1985, p. 2). Photography is a medium that offers many possibilities and can be used to communicate a variety of messages.

The camera has enlarged our world in space and time. It can enter the secret places of our civilizations, and it allows us to look closely at what is around us and maybe "see" it for the first time. It brings us closer to famous and important people. Beloff (1985) said, "We can all possess the icon" (p. 10) through a photograph; it gives evidence of personal experience and worth. Finally, pictures can show us things we might never be able to see otherwise; for example, the chambers of the heart or the victims of famine in Africa.

Photographs are an important part of all aspects of our culture, and they have strong powers of persuasion. As viewers, "we bring to a picture a whole set of personal and social associations" (Beloff, 1985, p. 18) and thereby give a photograph significant meaning.

As part of a teaching strategy, photographs have the *advantage* of being readily accessible through personal photo albums

(Gerace, 1989), books and magazines about photography, and general publications. They also can be produced by the faculty member and the students without too much difficulty. Photographs allow us to "stop the action" of a situation so we may study it very carefully. They often can be enlarged, duplicated, or made into slides to increase their accessibility to a group. Photography is a familiar and easily transportable art form; it also can make paintings, sculpture, and situations available for study at the faculty member's or students' convenience.

Photographs have some *disadvantages*. They may not capture the richness of a situation because they "stop the action" and record only a piece of total reality. Finding the "right" photograph, even at agencies that catalog collections for rental, can be time-consuming, and it can become quite costly to produce one's own photos and obtain the albums, frames, or slide carousels needed to store them properly.

In addition to personal collections, which convey growth and development, generational differences and interactions, and changes in social norms (e.g., dress), there are many excellent sources of photos. *Dust to Dust* (Heiden, 1992) is a photo book, with narrative, of a doctor's view of famine in Africa; *Epitaphs for the Living* (Howard, 1989) presents poignant photos of and words written by individuals with AIDS; and a special issue of *LIFE* magazine (The world . . . , 1990) was devoted to photos of children of all ages from around the world. *Aperture*, a journal, has excellent photos of people, situations, and communities throughout the world, as do *National Geographic, The New Yorker*, and the *Smithsonian* magazine. Browsing through bookstores and libraries may yield source books such as *A Way of Seeing* (Levitt, 1981), which presents photos of children from all cultures; *A Day in the Life of America* (Smolan & Cohen, 1986) and *An Album of the American Family Life* (1980), which depict various communities, cultures, and life situations.

Despite their disadvantages, photographs provide many opportunities for the teaching of nursing. An interesting exercise might inform students that 118 photographs were included in the Voyager interstellar spacecraft to illustrate Earth to extraterrestrials. Students might ponder or carry out a project answering the following question: If you were to include photographs about nurses and nursing in a time capsule, what would you include? Given the very personal meanings that individuals ascribe to photographs, the results of this exercise could be quite fascinating. Students' attitudes toward nursing, their understanding of the broad scope of nursing's influence, and the messages about nursing they would like to convey to others could be revealed through such an exercise. Photographs have the potential for providing fun and an exciting approach to teaching and learning nursing.

CONCLUSION

The arts and humanities are important elements in the preparation of an educated individual who is capable of addressing the complexity, ambiguity, and uncertainty of our world, which is characterized by unparalleled change and inhabited by billions of very unique individuals. Students of nursing benefit from interacting with the arts and humanities, not only through courses taught by experts in the fields of literature, fine arts, and film, but in nursing courses as well.

The registered nurses interviewed by Hagerty and Early (1993) noted that liberal education had expanded their minds, exposed them to different perspectives and ideas, helped them appreciate a "big picture," enhanced their self-awareness, and promoted their receptivity to the world. Sadly, many of these nurses commented that they were "unable to see the relevance of their liberal arts and science courses while in school and only came to appreciate content and perspectives after additional life and work experiences" (p. 154). Through the integration of the arts and humanities into nursing courses, students can be helped to see their relevance long before they graduate.

Nursing faculty are charged with the responsibility of preparing safe, competent practitioners who provide compassionate care. Although they may not be able to teach students to care, faculty can foster caring through personal and professional role modeling of caring behaviors and a genuine sensitivity to the uniqueness of others. The use of creative teaching strategies, including integrating the arts and humanities into nursing education, enhances students' understanding of who they are, what it means to be human, and how it feels to care.

Nurse educators can help students do more than merely tolerate liberal arts courses or observe "dead canvas or cold marble" (Nightingale). They can help students appreciate the intensity of life, the diversity of their fellow human beings, and the richness of the world around them by integrating the arts and humanities into the teaching and learning experiences they design. One does not need to be an expert in each of the areas of fine arts discussed here in order to use them to help students learn nursing concepts. What one *does* need, however, is an openness of mind, an appreciation of the art as well as the science of nursing, and a willingness to take risks and use new approaches to stimulate learning and a love of nursing.

REFERENCES

Adams, R. (1972). *Watership Down.* New York: Macmillan.

Allen, W. (Director). (1986). *Hannah and her sisters* [Film].

An album of the American family life. (1980). Radnor, PA: Sun Co.

Angus, D. (Ed.). (1962). *The best short stories of the modern age.* New York: Fawcett.

Armour, R. A., & Fuhrmann, B. S. (Eds.). (1989). *Integrating liberal learning and professional education* (New Directions for Teaching and Learning, No. 40). San Francisco: Jossey-Bass.

Bartol, G. M. (1986). Using the humanities in nursing education. *Nurse Educator, 11*(1), 21–23.

Beloff, H. (1985). *Camera culture.* New York: Basic Blackwell.

Boyer, E. (1987). *College: The undergraduate experience in America.* New York: Harper & Row.

Cardozo, N. B. (1992, March 22). Children's books (Review of *Journey*). *The New York Times,* 25.

Coles, R. (1978). *A festering sweetness: Poems of American people.* Pittsburgh, PA: University of Pittsburgh Press.

Conroy, C. (1976). *The great Santini.* Boston: Houghton Mifflin.

Curtis, M. H. (1985). Confronting an ancient dichotomy: A proposal for integrating liberal and professional education. *National Forum, 65*(3), 10-12.

Dickoff, J., & James, P. (1970). Beliefs and values: Bases for curriculum design. *Nursing Research, 19*(5), 415-426.

Donahue, M. P. (1988). *Nursing: The finest art.* St. Louis: Mosby.

Donaldson, S. (1983). Let us not abandon the humanities. *Nursing Outlook, 31*(1), 40-43.

Futrell, J. C. (1983). Learning leadership from *Watership Down. Human Development, 3*(4), 172-179.

Gerace, L. M. (1989). Using family photographs to explore life cycle changes. *Nursing & Health Care, 10*(5), 245-249.

Germain, C. P. (1986). Using literature to teach nursing. *Journal of Nursing Education, 25*(2), 84-86.

Gibran, K. (1973). *The prophet.* New York: Knopf.

Goldreich, G. (1977). What is death? The answers in children's books. *Hastings Center Report, 6*, 18-20.

Gustafson, M. B. (1979). Methods of teaching—Revisited. Try haiku. *The Journal of Continuing Education in Nursing, 10*(4), 59-60.

Hagerty, B., & Early, S. L. (1993). Registered nurses' perceptions of liberal education. *Journal of Nursing Education, 32*(4), 151-155.

Heiden, D. (1992). *Dust to dust.* Philadelphia: Temple University Press.

Hoshiko, B. (1985). Nursing diagnosis at the art museum. *Nursing Outlook, 33*(1), 32-36.

Howard, B. (1989). *Epitaphs for the living: Words and images in the time of AIDS.* Dallas, TX: Southern Methodist University Press.

Krysl, M. (1988). Existential moments of caring: Facets of nursing and social support. *Advances in Nursing Science, 10*(2), 12-17.

Krysl, M. (1989). *Midwife and other poems on caring.* New York: National League for Nursing.

Lee, R. T. (1986). The role of the arts in teaching effectively. *Educational Horizons, 64*(2), 62-66.

Levitt, H. (1981). *A way of seeing.* New York: Horizon Press.

Loden, K. C. (1989). Clinical experience at the museum of art. *Nurse Educator, 13*(3), 25-26.

MacLachlan, P. (1992). *Journey.* New York: Delacorte.

Matza, M. (1988, June 9). Checking out PBS classics. *The New York Times,* pp. 11, 4D.

Mukand, J. (1988). *Sutured words: Contemporary poetry about medicine.* Brookline, MA: Aviva Press.

Newell, L. J. (1989). The healing arts and the liberal arts in concert. In R. A. Armour & B. S. Fuhrmann (Eds.), *Integrating liberal learning and professional education* (New Directions for Teaching and Learning, No. 40) (pp. 67-76). San Francisco: Jossey-Bass.

Oiler, C. (1983). Nursing reality as reflected in poetry. *Perspectives in Psychiatric Care, 21*(3), 81-89.

Peck, M. L., & Jennings, S. (1989). Student perceptions of the links between nursing and the liberal arts. *Journal of Nursing Education, 28*(9), 406-414.

Peck, S. E. (1993). Monitoring student learning with poetry writing. *Journal of Nursing Education, 32*(4), 190-191.

Perrine, L. (Ed.). (1983). *Literature: Structure, sound, and sense* (4th ed.). New York: Harcourt.

Petrie, D. (Director). (1961). *A raisin in the sun* [Film].

Priest, R. R. (1970). The humanities in the nursing curriculum. In M. Q. Innis (Ed.), *Nursing education in a changing society* (pp. 184-189). Toronto: University of Toronto Press.

Read, H. (1968). *The meaning of art.* London: Faber & Faber.

Schier, F. (1988, February 14). Book review of "Painting as an art." *New York Times Book Review,* 13-14.

Smith, D. B. (1973). *A taste of blackberries.* New York: Crowell.

Smolan, R., & Cohen, D. (Project Directors). (1986). *A day in the life of America.* New York: Collins.

Text of Cheney's "Report to the President, the Congress, and the American People" on the humanities in America. (1988). *Chronicle of Higher Education, 35*(4), A17-A23.

The world of children. (1990, Spring). *LIFE,* special issue.

The volume library. (1982). Nashville, TN: Southwestern Co.

Wilson, H. S. (1974). A case for humanities in professional nursing education. *Nursing Forum, 12*(4), 406-417.

Wold, M., & Cykler, E. (1967). *An introduction to music and art in the western world.* Dubuque, IA: Brown.

Young-Mason, J. (1991). The Secret Sharer as a guide to compassion. *Nursing Outlook, 39*(2), 62-63.

Younger, J. B. (1990). Library works as a mode of knowing. *Image: Journal of Nursing Scholarship, 22,* 39-43.

7

Incorporating Multiple Modes of Awareness in Nursing Curriculum

Mary Koithan

*N*ursing pedagogy has long been debated in the United States. Educational standards and goals, curricular format, and classroom teaching methods have been extensively studied by nursing and educational researchers, discussed by discipline leaders, and changed frequently during the past 60 years (Bevis, 1988). Standardization of a nursing curriculum that concentrated on "training rather than education, on technique rather than understanding" at the associate and baccalaureate degree levels reached such a level of conformity and rigidity by the early 1980s that nursing leaders at the 1987 National League for Nursing Conference on Education and 1989 Wingspread Conference on Caring called for radical changes within the models for nursing curriculum development (*Curriculum revolution . . . ,* 1988, p. vii).

Sakalys and Watson (1986) proposed that the purpose of higher education is both epistemological and political (p. 92). Education should assist the learner in the pursuit of knowledge and reasoning skills. Furthermore, educational programs have social value in their response to societal needs and changing political environments. University graduates are individuals who are prepared to meet the needs of current society and to "think well." Yet, historically, it has been difficult to meld and harmonize these two seemingly divergent purposes within curricular development programs at the university level.

To address both epistemological and political concerns of professional education, nursing programs have undergone evolutionary changes in curriculum development throughout their history. Bevis (1988) noted five turns in nursing curriculum and traced the evolution of nursing education from a moral and ethical foundation during the Nightingale era to a technocratic, prescriptive model in the mid- to late 1900s. In recent years, nursing educators have been called to revolutionize the process of nursing education, to "depart from the old order" and create a "new public policy" for nursing and nursing education (Bevis, 1988; Watson, 1989). There is a renewed interest in harmonizing the epistemological call for education to support "thinking" and the political need for programs in higher education to continue to produce professional practitioners who will assist the citizenry in their search for health and care. Educational methods that are divergent from the currently used Tyler-type models are of profound interest to baccalaureate education program planners. Innovative teaching methods that emphasize (1) nursing's moral and social imperative to care for individuals and society, (2) creative and critical awareness, and (3) feminist learning principles need to be designed, used, tested, and evaluated within schools of nursing. The soul of nursing, the inner beauty of the nurse and the nursing student, again needs cultivation and awakening. It is time for nursing to revolutionize its educational programs, at the undergraduate and graduate levels, to consistently reflect nursing's philosophical, political, and epistemological beliefs and purposes.

THE PHILOSOPHY, EPISTEMOLOGY, AND POLITICS OF NURSING

Newman, Sime, and Corcoran-Perry (1991) identified three paradigmatic perspectives that have been and continue to be of use to the discipline of nursing. These orientations represent distinct and divergent ontological, epistemological, and metaphysical world-views that nursing uses to examine its phenomena of central interest, define its metaparadigmatic concepts, and develop theoretical perspectives for the discipline of nursing. Further, these world-views represent varied political and social commitments of the discipline. Nursing literature continues to provide examples of nursing's divergence in world-views with seemingly conflictual and inconsistent meanings of concepts and research methodologies used by the discipline. Yet, if individual programs of research, theory development, and education reflect a clear understanding as to the philosophical perspective represented, the discipline of nursing is enriched through the use of varied approaches to the nature of reality and the nature of knowing (Corcoran-Perry, 1992).

Many researchers who have contributed to the development of nursing science hold a view of science that is congruent with Carnap (1966) and is termed the natural science paradigm or the particulate–deterministic perspective (Newman et al., 1991). The ontological beliefs associated with the natural science or mechanistic paradigm include linear time (which exists separately from space), knowable reality (which is separate from historical and cultural contexts), and generalizable facts and laws (which exist separately from human beings) (Carnap, 1966; Grof, 1985; Tinkle & Beaton, 1983). Knowing occurs through a process of objectification, quantification, and reductionism of the subject to object (Carnap, 1966; Tinkle & Beaton, 1986). Consciousness is limited to living organisms and requires a highly developed neurological system.

Nursing has always been concerned about the person and his or her relation to other human beings and to the world. To this end, the value of the particulate–deterministic philosophical perspective to the discipline of nursing has been questioned. "Almost without exception the nurse authors, in talking about the goals and purposes of nursing, the content of nursing theory, and the criteria by which to evaluate nursing theory, emphasize the importance of sociohistorical or person–environment interaction. There is strong evidence of a deep commitment to nursing conceptualized in a relational sense" (Tinkle & Beaton, 1983, p. 589). The use of the particulate–deterministic model leaves nursing conceptualizations isolated, dichotomized, and dehumanized. Nursing's epistemology has been widely divergent from its ontological beliefs about the reality of the world. Therefore, alternative paradigmatic perspectives viewed as more consistent with nursing's commitments, beliefs, and moral imperatives have evolved.

Newman et al. (1991) identified the interactive–integrative perspective as a natural evolutionary response to the criticisms of the natural science or particulate–deterministic philosophy of science. Although more consistent with nursing's beliefs and values, the interactive model does not address nursing's beliefs and concerns in totality. "Phenomena are viewed as having multiple, interrelated parts in relation to a specific context . . . ; and change . . . is a function of antecedent factors and probabilistic relationships" (Newman et al., 1991, p. 4). This perspective has been used within nursing research, theory development, and clinical practice since the early 1960s. Many of the current theories of nursing assume this integrative perspective.

Yet, nursing's values of holism, unidirectional change, and unpredictability are again not fully reflected by the integrative scientific world-view. Nursing scholars often critique theorists who decry a lack of commitment to holistic beliefs as articulated within conceptual frameworks, health as an evolutionary process, and the change as the way of life (Mitchell & Cody, 1992; Parse, 1987). Language frequently found in nursing literature reflects a lack of clarity as to the discipline's values, beliefs, and philosophical perspective. Therefore, a third philosophical perspective is entertained as necessary for the discipline of nursing.

Newman et al. (1991) proposed that this third scientific world-view "is essential to the full explication of the discipline" of nursing (p. 5). The unitary–transformative paradigmatic perspective represents a "significant shift" in the ontological, epistemological, and metaphysical beliefs about this world (p. 4). Newman et al. (1991) again offered that the scientific tradition essential to the mission of caring and nursing is neither the mechanistic nor the integrative approach, but rather is the unitary-transformative perspective.

Many authors suggest the same emergence of a transcendent, unitary-transformative paradigm that will provide a convergent view of science consistent with the values of nursing as a professional discipline (Giorgi, 1970; Grof, 1985; Newman et al., 1991; Stember & Hester, 1990; Watson, 1985, 1992). Among the emergent paradigm's several titles are: transpersonal, holonomic, and unitary-transformative (Bohm, 1980; Giorgi, 1970; Grof, 1985; Newman et al., 1991). This perspective can be described as holistic and concerned with the unique human phenomenon as experienced by the individual. A closed attitude toward phenomenal interpretation is rejected by human science; an "engaged" and open approach to the analysis of phenomenal experience is the desired outcome (Giorgi, 1970). Paternalistic attitudes of categorization, reductionism, and manipulation are inconsistent with the new world-view (Watson, 1985b). All phenomena are viewed as "unified self-organizing fields embedded into a larger self-organizing field . . . which is identified by pattern" and unitary interaction with the larger whole (Newman et al., 1991). Change is characterized as unidirectional, unpredictable movement leading to greater complexity in organization, an "unfolding" (Newman et al., 1991, p. 4).

The ontological beliefs of the transcendent, unitary-transformative paradigm include dedication to holistic human beings, multiple realities, idiographic as well as nomothetic information concerning humans and the world, and unique as well as generalizable understanding about the phenomena of human concern. The nature of reality is described as an unbroken and coherent whole that is involved in an unending process of change—the "holomovement" (Bohm, 1980). Space-time boundaries may be transcended in human experience to include spiritual identification of relationships with the totality of the universe, the collective consciousness, or the totality of life on this planet. Nursing's inclusion of beliefs from the unitary-transformative as a probable philosophical perspective necessarily leads to changes in the discipline's definition of its metaparadigm, development of its theories, and approach to its epistemological and political commitments.

Nursing's moral and social imperative subsequent to the inclusion of the unitary-transformative perspective is based on the ontological commitment to care as a central phenomenon for the discipline of nursing. Nursing is the "study of caring in the human health experience" (Newman et al., 1991). Caring is defined as "helping another person to grow and actualize himself. . . . It is a way of relating to someone that involves mutual trust, resulting in a transformative relationship for both the one caring and the one cared for" (Mayeroff, 1971, pp. 1-2; Noddings, 1984). Caring entails attending to the abstract and the concrete, the local as well as the global concerns of people (Benner, 1989).

Caring mandates commitment to others, commitment to the reembodiment of the recipient of care, and respect for human qualities. No longer can nursing be totally concerned with and subsumed by the technocratic, curative aspects of the current health care system. A utilitarian approach to health care and a beneficent, paternalistic approach to the care of individuals are no longer the moral imperatives of the discipline of nursing (Gadow, 1989). The person as a whole—a participatory, growing, experiential being—becomes the moral focus of human caring. Caring and nursing rejoice in the unique and subjective.

Caring, thus described, becomes the ontological stance of nursing (Watson, 1992). Caring and its inherent values of person, knowledge, relational patterning, and consciousness become a way of "being in the world," the ultimate reality. Caring cannot be reduced to technique; rather, it informs our very nature, our soul, our self. Care gives value to humanness and leads to transformation of the human spirit (Watson, 1992).

Nursing's commitment to care as the foundation for its political and social mandates and its adoption of multiple philosophical perspectives, including the unitary-transformative world-view, necessarily guide nursing's epistemological convictions. "I must know many things if I am to care" (Mayeroff, 1971, p. 13). Caring requires attentiveness, pattern recognition, honesty, openness, courage, and knowledge. One cannot care in a vacuum. The nurse must be aware of knowledge that is available; be alert to meanings conveyed through written, verbal, and nonverbal discourse; discern which information is necessary to the care of the human being, given this time and space; and implement the necessary interventions to support and facilitate health seeking. Knowledge is acquired through multiple modes of awareness; they include empirical, ethical, personal, and aesthetic patterns of recognition and knowing (Carper, 1978). Empirical information is necessary to explain the unfolded nature of reality, which lends itself well to quantitative as well as qualitative data collection. The body physical, and nursing's commitment to it, is not to be neglected for other areas of interest (Watson, 1992).

Moral knowledge stems from the discipline's ethical and moral commitment to care. Watson (1990) called us to a "wide-awakeness" where moral passion becomes informed through caring as the reflection of life and life forces, which is not simply technical correctness. Moral knowledge is developed through a process of existential caring that involves honesty, trust, humility, and hope (Carper, 1978, p. 15). This process of pattern recognition leads to the acknowledgment and understanding of the patient as person, "beyond categorical recognition," and to the perception of the individual as a whole (Carper, 1978, p. 15).

Personal knowledge is best described as intuition. A growing body of quantitative research is acknowledging the use of intuition within the clinical care of patients (Baumann & Deber, 1989; Prescott, Dennis, & Jacox, 1987; Rew, 1988). Benner (1984) indicated that the use and value of personal knowledge greatly increase in the expert nurse. "Personal knowledge is concerned with the knowing, encountering, and actualizing of the concrete, individual self" (Carper, 1978). Cultivation and acute listening to the inner self form a process that must be rediscovered among nursing students.

Aesthetic knowledge is particularly important to the understanding of concepts and meanings that are not easily translated into verbal and written communication. Often, meaning is lost in the word through which the concept is communicated. Understanding, however, is augmented through arts such as poetry, painting, sculpture, music, or photography. The difference primarily is one of perception rather than recognition. Perception unifies ends and means leading to understanding and ultimately to action (Carper, 1978).

Watson (1989) called for a revolution in nursing's social policy agenda, based on human care and caring. With the identification of care as nursing's ontological stance and social purpose, changes would be sought in the current health care system, the current domestic policy of the United States, and the current economic-technological models of society. Nursing's social and political mission would finally be consistent with its philosophical perspectives. The dramatic paradigmatic shift in nursing's philosophical perspectives and the revolution in nursing's social and political policy, coupled with changing epistemological beliefs, would signify a convergence in fundamental tenets of nursing and serve to direct the future of nursing education.

Nursing's epistemological and political purposes in education converge within a context of the transformative paradigm, human care and caring, and multiple ways of knowing. Simply stated, it is in the best interests of politics and nursing's social mandate that caregivers "think well." Nursing curricula must address both epistemological and political purposes in the education of future generations of nurses. In an environment of revolutionizing health and nursing care, nurses must think well to care.

REVOLUTIONIZING BACCALAUREATE EDUCATION IN NURSING

Current undergraduate-level programs in nursing need to be examined and critically reviewed so that they consistently reflect nursing's philosophical, epistemological, and social beliefs and values. Radical changes in nursing's curricular structure and teaching methodologies follow from the adoption of beliefs and values that embrace personal knowing, aesthetic awareness, holism, fluidity, human caring and process as the desired end product, humanism, and personal value and worth. Tyler-type curricular models need to be abandoned so that students are not treated as products of an industrialized educational setting—that is, "We must change our metaphor" (Bevis, 1988, p. 47). Educational programs need to be revolutionized. Students must be educated in the principles and processes of thinking well so that care and caring might be fostered among professional nursing graduates.

Teaching methods and teacher–learner roles must also be revolutionized. Bevis (1988) suggested the replacement of item learning, directive learning, and rational learning. These methods of learning, currently used in professional nursing education, foster technical training rather than critical and creative reasoning/thinking. Syntactical, contextual, and inquiry learning methods promote innovative teaching-learning dialog between faculty and students and educate rather than train the nursing student (Bevis, 1988, p. 44). Students are encouraged, through a variety of teaching-learning techniques that incorporate syntactical, contextual, and inquiry learning methods, to find patterning and meaning in the concepts introduced. Personal understanding is enhanced through insight and "intuitive leaps" (Bevis, 1988). The language of nursing's moral commitment to caring, to humanistic, altruistic values, and to relationship building is conveyed to students. Finally, students are encouraged to develop creative methods of inquiry, idea generation, and dream visualizations. Students thus become liberated to achieve maximally rather than minimally through the nursing curriculum.

Teaching methods and the teacher-learner relationship would be altered significantly with the adoption of radically different learning methods. "To mount our revolution we must dispense with the view of the teacher as an information-giver either in the classroom or in the practicum" (Bevis, 1988, p. 46). Rather, the instructor becomes facilitator, role model, and nurturer. Group projects and discussion replace lecture as teaching method. Aesthetics, personal journaling, critical writing, and self-appraisal replace objective testing and quantified evaluation methods. The classroom becomes a safe context within which discovery, creativity, and questioning are welcome.

Through dramatic curricular revolution, nursing education will provide professional education that is consistent with the philosophical, epistemological, and moral beliefs of the discipline. Educational purposes will finally converge so that graduates of nursing programs fulfill nursing's social and political agenda of caring in the human health experience through a process of creative and critical thinking, personal valuing, and professional courage.

Implementation of a Caring Curriculum

Revolution in nursing education will most likely proceed in a steplike fashion wherein individual faculty members or individual schools of nursing examine curricular structure, individual courses, and individual teaching styles. Mandated changes and the unified replacement of the Tyler-type curricular model with another similar structure would lead to institutionalization rather than the revolution and creativity that we seek (Bevis, 1988; Watson, 1988). Therefore, individual creativity and innovation need to be encouraged and nurtured within the community of nursing educators and scholars.

When curricular revolution occurs, as evidenced by a shift in faculty awareness and commitments to alternative philosophical perspectives for the discipline of nursing, individual nursing educators are encouraged to revise courses to be consistent with changing ontological and epistemological tenets of the unitary-transformative paradigm. A caring curriculum need not be adopted throughout the entire nursing program for the students to be given the opportunity to experience nursing's changing beliefs. Indeed, the unitary-transformative educational perspective encourages divergence in thought and individual evaluation of multiple possibilities so that personal selections and choices are based on the meaning and explanatory power derived from the perspective.

When the philosophical basis of education is consistent with the philosophy, epistemology, and social agenda of nursing, the presentation style, student evaluation methods, and course objectives/subjectives need to be examined and redesigned to incorporate multiple modes of awareness. These modes would include aesthetics and intuition; personal choice based on individual student illumination of meaning; and critical thinking based on an expanded definition of human awareness. Courses that embody the tenets of a changing perspective on human awareness (defined to include aesthetic knowing) would be designed to be interactive rather than directive. Class work would be based on discovery of relationships rather than memorization of fact. Class topics would follow general outlines, but class time would be planned to be participatory and lectures would be minimal. These techniques would incorporate nursing's commitment to multiple modes of awareness, including empirics, aesthetics, and personal ways of knowing.

Classroom presentation methods should emphasize the power of these multiple modes of awareness. Art, photography, music, aromas, and metaphor in the classroom create new dimensions of understanding within students and validate the potential use of aesthetics and creative expression in patient teaching–learning and caring instances. Students should be encouraged to incorporate personal events into the classroom work, thereby dramatically increasing their understanding of the human health experience through intuition or personal knowing modalities and emphasizing the diverse nature of human learning and life.

Generally, topics for class discussion should be structured so that minimal new fact/knowledge is imparted each week. Each class should build on the past weeks, to allow whole conceptual relationships to be visualized by semester's end. Although the transition from fact to experience in the classroom is difficult for those who categorize and analyze the details of every operation, students need to begin to appreciate the profession of nursing as a whole and the impact of one concept on the nature of others. Nursing's philosophical beliefs of holism and increasing diversity need to become manifest within the curriculum. These tenets awaken within the personal experience of each student and form a basis for lifelong learning and caring.

The reading assignments for class, collected from philosophical papers, novels, poetry, and texts, should reflect a commitment to nursing's diverse epistemological beliefs. Aesthetic appreciation and knowing can be demonstrated to students through the use of poetry, metaphor, and storytelling. Novels that have been used in nursing curricula with successful result include *One* (Bach, 1988), *The Metamorphosis* (Kafka, 1974), *A Reckoning* (Sarton, 1978), and *The Birth of a Grandfather* (Sarton, 1989). Poems by Krysl (1989), Whitman (1959), Angelou (1974), and Frost (1964) present vibrant images that become etched in students' memory. Students should be asked to interrelate concepts by using aesthetic expression found in their own environment. Their personal knowing can be enhanced by guiding students to always read critically, to relate what is read to their personal experience, and to journal their impressions and feelings regarding the reading assignments.

Within a curriculum emphasizing multiple modes of awareness, critical thinking process methodologies that proceed strictly along the deductive-reductionistic pathway are antithetical to fundamental beliefs and are viewed as counterproductive. Nursing faculty have historically identified nursing process and disciplined inquiry as the primary methods for critical thinking within the discipline of nursing. However, nursing faculty should encourage the use of multiple modalities that facilitate critical thinking (philosophical analysis, moral reasoning, personal awareness, and aesthetic discovery) and a more flexible definition of clinical problem solving and disciplined inquiry. Creativity and individual styles of problem solving should be celebrated and recognized as the desired outcome of any revolutionized curriculum.

Evaluation methods for the reformed classroom would encourage students to explore meanings, develop cognitive relationships among the concepts discussed, and personally discover within their own lives patterns that are affected or will become affected by the meanings found in the ideas examined during class work. Assignments should reflect creative ideas about nursing care within the human health experience by assimilating the empirical, aesthetic, moral, and personal knowledge of each student. A "creative project," wherein students prepare and submit presentations that aesthetically describe major nursing concepts, might be used as one method of student evaluation. This aesthetically creative process assists in the development of personal and aesthetic knowing and an appreciation for the "Aha!" phenomenon.

Creative expression is necessary for the discipline of nursing, but nursing students also need to be able to clearly communicate their thoughts in writing, appreciate the empirical and moral ways of coming to know and understand, and critically investigate the meaning of their beliefs and values by employing syntactical and inquiry learning. Thought or opinion papers are vehicles for evaluating students' ability to participate in analytical reasoning. These papers also integrate personal, empirical, and moral ways of knowing through the processes of critical analysis and justification.

Thought papers seek to uncover ideas and views that students have regarding the profession and discipline of nursing, their personal philosophy of nursing care, and their understanding of theoretical perspectives covered during the entire course. Student papers should be evaluated for their justification, clarity and consistency in thought and writing, and evidence of an ability to use the vocabulary and expression introduced in the class.

The incorporation of alternatives to traditional student evaluation does not necessarily mandate a complete abandonment of examinations or nursing process papers. Rather, adoption of changing philosophical and epistemological beliefs requires a transformation in the faculty's approach to the teaching–learning and evaluation processes. Examination styles that incorporate methods of justification enhance student learning and provide greater depth of evaluation by the instructor. Nursing process papers need not follow prescribed formats or include standardized intervention modalities. Conferencing, rather than grading, may be used as an alternative method of evaluation, to facilitate resolution of creative problems and to increase the appreciation of student–faculty individualism, which is highly valued in a reformed curriculum.

An Environment of Care and Creativity

When the commitment to care is the ontological stance of nursing, the educational environment must model respect, mutuality, and courageous trust. During the times when small groups meet, students should be encouraged to leave the classroom for a more ideal setting—out-of-doors, in the library, or wherever the group feels most comfortable. This freedom in movement helps to cultivate trust in purpose, the development of more honest feelings and conclusions, and greater creativity. During student or group sharing, participants should be allowed to choose the seating and the presentation style most comfortable for them. Flexibility should be the byword of class work.

Writing and empirical presentation styles should also be allowed to be flexible. Nursing process can be written in any format. Although this proves discomforting at first, most students evolve a style that meets their own visualization needs and patterns of recognition. Papers can be written in essay or outline format, or relayed through storytelling and metaphor. In this method of student evaluation, those who are more traditionally focused excel as comfortably as others who are not.

The questioning or seminar format helps to establish a more open and safer haven for students than the traditional classroom. Class time that is dedicated solely to questions and problem solving provides everyone an opportunity to air grievances, state difficulties, and exchange information. If this planned time is scheduled at the beginning of class, problems and questions are never left unresolved because of lack of time and/or energy. All opinions are valued explicitly through comments from faculty and students. All questions are considered thoughtfully through mutual sharing and learning. No comment, opinion, or question, no matter the content or tenor of presentation, is denigrated or ignored.

Student achievements are readily acknowledged by faculty and student peers. Although hesitant at first, students quickly find the "standing ovation" a great way to reward others and self for their accomplishments of the past week. This idea was generated through discussion at the University of Colorado Health Sciences Center's School of Nursing by faculty who taught in the baccalaureate program (Watson, 1992). The last five minutes of class is spent in this activity, so that the class always ends on a positive, inspirational note on which the students and faculty can focus for the entire week. By semester's end, even if time is short, students are usually requesting that we not forget the standing ovation and often opt to cut discussion short so that there is ample time to applaud their friends.

CONCLUSION

Curriculum revolution is currently nursing education's call to arms. Nursing leadership summons educators to depart from the old-order, Tyler-type curricular models that concentrate on training nursing students and, instead, embark on a creative journey to nursing education within a framework that addresses nursing's philosophical, epistemological, and social beliefs and purposes. Students then become educated to think well in order to lead the implementation of nursing's social and political mandate to care.

New educational models must reflect nursing's commitment to holistic persons who come to know and understand through multiple modes of awareness. Environmental structures will take on new meaning as nursing extends its philosophical and moral beliefs regarding care, person, and environment to the classroom. Educational styles and teacher–learner relationships will be redefined by examination through a lens of caring and feminist values. Students will be introduced to nursing in a manner that is consistent with our values of human dignity, self-worth, and care, thus enhancing the inner beauty and pride of nurses and nursing. Given this belief in the future and in the beauty and worth of self, and if taught well to think creatively, aesthetically, and critically, nurses could lead the way to a national health care policy focused on caring and caring, human advancement and evolution, and health, healing, and wholeness.

REFERENCES

Angelou, M. (1974). *Gather together in my name.* New York: Random House.

Bach, R. (1988). *One.* New York: Dell.

Baumann, A., & Deber, R. (1989). The limits of decision analysis for rapid decision making in ICU nursing. *Image: The Journal of Nursing Scholarship, 21*(2), 69-71.

Benner, P. (1984). *From novice to expert: Excellence and power in clinical nursing practice.* Menlo Park, CA: Addison-Wesley.

Benner, P. (1989). The moral dimensions of caring. In *Knowledge about care and caring* (pp. 5-17). Kansas City, MO: American Academy of Nursing.

Bevis, E. (1988). New directions for a new age. In *Curriculum revolution: Mandate for change* (pp. 27-52). New York: National League for Nursing.

Bohm, D. (1980). *Wholeness and the implicate order*. London: Routledge & Kegan Paul.

Carnap, R. (1966). *Philosophical foundations of physics*. New York: Basic Books.

Carper, B. (1978). Fundamental patterns of knowing in nursing. *Advances in Nursing Science, 1*(1), 13-23.

Corcoran-Perry, S. (1992). Personal communication. University of Minnesota, Minneapolis.

Curriculum revolution: Mandate for change. (1988). New York: National League for Nursing.

Frost, R. (1964). *Complete poems of Robert Frost*. New York: Holt, Rinehart and Winston.

Gadow, S. (1989). The advocacy covenant: Care as clinical subjectivity. In *Knowledge about care and caring* (pp. 33-40). Kansas City, MO: American Academy of Nursing.

Giorgi, A. (1970). *Psychology as a human science*. New York: Harper & Row.

Grof, S. (1985). *Beyond the brain*. Albany, NY: SUNY Press.

Kafka, F. (1974). *The metamorphosis*. New York: Bantam Books.

Krysl, M. (1989). *Midwife and other poems on caring*. New York: National League for Nursing.

Mayeroff, M. (1971). *On caring*. New York: Harper & Row.

Mitchell, G., & Cody, W. (1992). Nursing knowledge and human science: Ontological and epistemological considerations. *Nursing Science Quarterly, 5*(2), 54-61.

Newman, M., Sime, A., & Corcoran-Perry, S. (1991). The focus of the discipline of nursing. *Advances in Nursing, 14*(1), 1-14.

Noddings, N. (1984). *Caring: A feminist approach to ethics and moral education*. Berkeley: University of California Press.

Parse, R. (1987). *Nursing science: Major paradigms, theories, and critiques*. Philadelphia: Saunders.

Prescott, P., Dennis, K., & Jacox, A. (1987). Clinical decision making of staff nurses. *Image: The Journal of Nursing Scholarship, 19*(2), 56-62.

Quinn, J. (1989). The Haelen effect. *Nursing and Health Care, 10*(10), 552-557.

Rew, L. (1988). Intuition in decision-making. *Image: The Journal of Nursing Scholarship, 20*(3), 150-154.

Sakalys, J., & Watson, J. (1986). Professional education: Post-baccalaureate education for professional nursing. *Journal of Professional Nursing,* 91-97.

Sarton, M. (1978). *A reckoning.* New York: Norton.

Sarton, M. (1989). *The birth of a grandfather.* New York: Norton.

Smith, J. (1983). *The idea of health.* New York: Teachers College Press.

Stember, M., & Hester, N. (1990). Research strategies for developing nursing as the science of human care. In N. Chaska, *The nursing profession* (pp. 165-172). St. Louis: Mosby.

Tinkle, M., & Beaton, J. (1983). Toward a new view of science: Implications for nursing research. *Advances in Nursing, 5*(2), 27-36.

Watson, J. (1985a). *Nursing: The philosophy and science of caring.* Boulder: The University of Colorado Press.

Watson, J. (1985). *Nursing: Human science and human care.* Norwalk, CT: Appleton-Century-Crofts.

Watson, J. (1988). Human caring as moral context for nursing education. *Nursing and Health Care, 9*(8), 423-425.

Watson, J. (1989). Human caring: A public agenda. In *Knowledge about care and caring* (pp. 41-48). Kansas City, MO: American Academy of Nursing.

Watson, J. (1990). Caring knowledge and informed moral passion. *Advances in Nursing Science, 13*(1), 15-23.

Watson, J. (1992, January). *Theory in human care nursing.* Symposium conducted at the University of Colorado Health Sciences Center, Boulder.

Whitman, W. (1959). *Complete poetry and prose.* Boston: Houghton Mifflin.

8

Narrative in Nursing Practice and Education

Toni M. Vezeau

The essential character of, say, pedagogy is always "yet-to-be-decided," not because of some lack of effort or lack of moral courage, but because children keep coming.

David W. Jardine

*N*arrative (in this context, creative fiction) is a product of an aesthetic process that attempts to bridge subjective and objective stances to the world by reversing the primary Western focus on the general. Science, mirroring the dominant culture, has not always effectively served certain populations, such as women, children, and minorities. Concerns have been exteriorly defined, research methods have looked for the most general response, and information has been generalized outside of the demographics of the data source.

Narrative can focus on particular responses to health and transition and, therefore, can give a voice where previously none was heard. There is considerable caution toward embracing the arts and humanities as serious inquiry, however. The very development of science has been to supplant story and the implied bias of the individual as a path to knowledge.

The purpose of this chapter is to clarify where narrative might fit with nursing education and nursing practice. Past strategies for the inclusion of the humanities have been only partially successful. The goal here (and elsewhere in this book) is to provide a discussion of how nursing might begin to develop approaches more in keeping with the nature of narrative as aesthetic process and product.

READING NARRATIVE

Nursing educators are becoming increasingly interested in the use of narrative for the discussion of values and differences in the experience of health. With the mandate, in many nursing programs, to incorporate the humanities into what are primarily scientific curricula, nursing educators have used narrative to aid in teaching the ethical component of nursing care. Nursing clinicians have been using narrative as an avenue for portrayal of unique experiences and nuances of nursing care for individuals. Because narrative is based in exploration of particular situations, it provides sharp contrast to the scientific research and theory that currently inform nursing.

Glenn Webster, a philosopher of science with a history of involvement in nursing, encouraged nursing not to view itself as a science (1990). Nursing is a profession that draws on the sciences, but, in doing so, it risks an overly narrow perspective.

Should nursing be supporting sciences in the traditional sense, or would it be more helpful . . . for nursing to support certain types of history and case studies, perhaps new branches of philosophy? . . . Nursing needs much richer sources in literature and philosophy than presently exist.

Should the research effort and funds of nursing support such endeavors as the writing of a new genre of short story and novel focusing on the experience of individuals and their families with health problems? Would it not be useful to nursing to have new work . . . expounding and developing the concept of caring? (Webster, 1990, p. 15)

Sally Gadow, a philosopher of nursing who has strongly supported the use of narrative in nursing education, agreed:

Am I suggesting that nursing is not a science? Yes, because it is a country, a region of experience. There are sciences that help, just as an Arctic explorer is helped by understanding principles of hypothermia, although the methods of its prevention must be learned through local knowledge . . . . Nursing is a world—in which people live and know. What do we know? We know how to attempt a "safe and honorable passage" through the endless dimensions that it presents. Not every passage will be safe, for patient or for nurse. There are risks; there must be. The stakes are high. It is life that is involved, not the study of life. (Gadow, 1990a, p. 10)

Gadow (1985, 1990a) considers narrative valuable in an education process that will help us encounter examples of a "'safe and honorable passage.'"

Nurse educators and clinicians have generally been schooled in the scientific realm and may not understand how narrative is different from science. There are some indications in scholarly nursing literature that narrative is misunderstood and used in ways that resemble research studies or theory (Bartol, 1989a).

Younger (1990), who supports the power of narrative to explore meaning and context in health, points to several stories, the biblical Book of Job, and Tolstoy's *The Death of Ivan Ilych* as having specific meaning for nursing students. The story of Job shows that bad things happen to good people, and Ivan Ilych teaches us that all persons search for meaning in illness. My disappointment is her approach is not explained by these being inadequate stories. They have persisted, and many persons have found great meaning in them. The problem I find is that Younger seems to support these stories not based on their power to evoke, but as tropes—figures of speech with definitive meaning. This story means this, that story means that. The reader remains an outsider to the story. There can be little engagement when the meaning is predetermined.

Similarly, Young-Mason (1988) advocated literature as a vehicle to help students understand moral decision making and saw classical Greek literature as capable of teaching suffering and compassion to all students:

> *The tragic figures display ideal morals and weaknesses and, since they come from another culture and time, it is possible to identify with them in a detached way that allows us to remember their plight and the actions they took, and to feel that their blunders as well as their courageous deeds are possible for us. (p. 299)*

Young-Mason encouraged students to:

> *. . . think of the literary figures as archetypes and to look for similarities between the characters and health care professionals in their reactions to and behavior toward the disfigured and difficult patient. [Students] are urged to dissect the reasons for the difficult patient's attitudes and actions. (pp. 299-300)*

Young-Mason's goal is to reach certitude with detachment, suggesting a scientific approach to education through narrative:

> *Beliefs and values can thus be defined and shared without personal revelation of either the student or the teacher. A safe, common ground is thus provided by working through and sharing a universal tragedy. (p. 300)*

In the field of education, the use of narrative has not always been treated benevolently, even by its advocates. Jardine and Clandinin (1987) seriously critiqued the usual approach to narrative—a form of "this means that." When texts or teachers propose themselves as sources of expertise, use of narrative does not seek to explore. It is as prescriptive as the control paradigm of traditional science. Jardine and Clandinin (1987) warned:

This, for us, gives teaching as storytelling the potential to be even more dangerous than the dominant model since it appears to remedy what it, in fact, reinforces. (p. 476)

If nursing is to thoroughly engage narrative in nursing education and practice, we must be careful to take an approach that is consistent with its metaphorical nature, instead of an approach that entails certainty or even probability. Narrative requires a pedagogical stance that is radically different from science.

Plausibility Is Not Generalizable

Both Younger and Younger-Mason assumed that the stories referenced in their articles are plausible to all readers. This assumption is incorrect. Plausibility cannot be determined for the reader.

A Martian nurse may not see Sophocles' plays as believable because cultural differences may make the context and plot unbelievable. Likewise, there is no reason to believe that a story chosen for a classroom discussion will seem plausible to all students. This is not because the student is deficient in "getting it." The dominant culture remains Greco-Roman and so those of us who belong to the hegemonic culture and share a similar context with the characters will more likely see such a story as plausible.

The assumption that plausibility can be generalizable recreates the fallacy in literary criticism that the development of a canon of meritorious stories is worthwhile to guide use of narrative. A literary canon implies that if a story is written well enough, it will be believable to all readers across place and time.

"This great book," "this worthless book," the same book is called by both names. Praise and blame alike mean nothing. No, delightful as the pastime of measuring may be, it is the most futile of all occupations, and to submit to the decrees of the measurers, the most servile of attitudes. So long

as you write what you wish to write, that is all that matters;
and whether it matters for ages or only for hours, nobody
can say. (Woolf, 1929, p. 185)

The same can be said of reading what one wants to read.

The establishment of an ethical canon of narrative ignores culture and the role of the reader in the creation of narrative meaning. Reading lists can be diverse in cultural backgrounds and styles (Bartol, 1989a). Nurse educators and clinicians would do well to look beyond classical literature and consider the inclusion of popular fiction as well. Even then, some stories will not speak to everyone in a group, even with additional cognitive information. There can be no exemplar stories to teach ethics in nursing. Readers ally themselves to specific stories based on an internal assessment of fit.

Cocreation of Meaning

In a similar vein, educators cannot assume that a story has a certain predetermined meaning or objective truth. Trustworthy fiction will necessarily lead to debate over meaning and will result in a multiplicity of interpretations. Those using narrative should hope to broaden the awareness of readers about their world and not dictate any particular interpretation of a story. Vitz (1990), an educational psychologist, stated that there is danger of indoctrination when the use of stories involves direct teaching of particular ethical content. Young-Mason wants to teach compassion to students by drawing on so-called classical themes literature. This may be appropriate in a literature class, but is it appropriate for nurses studying human experience?

There is no merit in agreement with the teacher concerning what a story means. There is no merit in the emulation of characters, "to feel that their blunders as well as their courageous deeds are possible for us" (Young-Mason, 1988, p. 229). There is a risk of narrative becoming catechism in such an educational approach.

A story teaches possibilities. It can never be generalizable explanation; it is solely exploration and never prescribes.

Full Engagement with Story

Both Younger and Young-Mason suggested one virtue of using narrative: Detachment from the emotional content of a story is possible. I suggest that this is not possible or desirable. Parker (1990), a nurse who also supports narrative in the development of an ethic of care, saw the engagement possible through narrative as essential to nursing education:

> *The strength of nursing is linked to nurses' refusal to adopt an impartial, detached posture in response to moral conflict. (p. 39)*

Banks, a prolific writer in the field of literature and health, would prefer that, to challenge the reader, ethicists concentrate not only on the content of a story but on its emotive power. Banks (1990) stated that drama is the primary mover within literature and is a "natural ally" to ethicists (p. 230). Ethical behavior is always, in the context of conflict, rife with emotion; for this reason, narrative is superb for ethical discussion.

> *Drama also serves clinical ethicists by demonstrating the intimate relationship between the meaning of a play and the reaction of an audience on any given day. After all, a play is not merely the words written on the page any more than an ethical decision consists solely of the language in which it is expressed. A play changes with each audience. As audience members respond to what they are able to hear that day, the actors in turn change their emphases. Thus, drama is constantly reinventing itself in response to the needs of its collaborators. What it gives up in terms of perfection, it gains in terms of humanity. (pp. 230-231)*

The power of narrative is that it moves us not only to think and evaluate, but to live in a special place, smelling the smells and feeling the full impact of human experience. It is important that nursing not ignore or downplay the emotive impact of story. Although it provides a place to live, a meeting place, that does not mean that this place is always safe. When a reader fully engages a story, a flood of personal experiences can be unleashed, triggered by the story's power. Readers will also vicariously experience new situations. This will surely disturb us—particularly in nursing, where we live within the range of human suffering.

The purpose of using narrative is not to provide easily analyzable archetypes and tropes for students to gain theoretical knowledge of human conflict in a safe and detached manner. Doing so reduces narrative to data.

> . . . when science tries to comprehend a world of experience wholly outside that of the scientist . . . the result is eventually the dismissal of local narratives . . . "Because the narrative cannot be reduced to a form that lends itself to a summary. [The writers'] words are too hard to turn into numbers." (Gadow, 1990b, p. 8, quoting Lopez, 1989, p. 270)

Narrative is intended to thoroughly engage people not only with a particular story but with their own lives (Bartol, 1989a, 1989b). Scientific education often leads persons to disengage from their own lives; they become disembodied practitioners who cannot care. Narrative can bring them home, in a context in which they need to be most human: ethical conflict.

The Focus of Narrative: The Reader, Not the Story

The focus of the use of story is, ultimately, not the story itself but the reader. Stone (1985), a poet and cardiologist who teaches literature and medicine, explained this approach:

> We begin with the art . . . but before very long we find ourselves discussing, not only the art, but our own lives as well. The art, the literature, has become a catalyst. The fact is, it's much easier, much less discomfiting, for any of us to talk about a novel than it is to talk about our lives, which is

what actually happens: we find ourselves recalling our own patients, our own illnesses, our own reactions to the practice of medicine. . . . In an encounter with art, the first and last curriculum is ourselves. *(1985, p. 8)*

Narrative as a method of inquiry for nursing can lead to a type of knowledge that is contextual and retains the mystery and complexity of human experience. Narrative is not a foreign country that we need to keep suspect; it is where we as humans normally live.

Perhaps this is the area in which clinicians have made best use of narratives. My experience in reading groups is that this uncovering of self and self-stories is allowed and encouraged. The discussion that is provoked by stories is the prime benefit to practicing nurses. In some instances, stories can be made available for private reading and personal reflection. Most often, I have used the stories in groups and meetings with families, students, and staff as a springboard for discussion about elusive aspects of interaction and subjective responses to health and transition.

Aoki (1991) discussed practitioners' attempts to understand teaching through story. Rarely do we *really listen* to each other's stories. The reading of stories and the dialogue that becomes inevitable afterward beckon new stories. If we value this emergence of new stories—if we are listened to—we flourish. If we learn to listen to simple speech about experiences, we can hear the "unsaid . . . something that he or she neither wants or dares to say. He/she may even make such implications by saying nothing" (Aoki, 1991, p. 6).

Expansive Quality of Story in the Discussion of a Category.   A story expands the meaning of what was previously thought to be understood. It bears a "family resemblance" that calls for further investigation (Jardine, 1992, p. 55). Narrative is not engaged in order to "get to the bottom of things" or to "hit the nail on the head"—the essence. If it were, after the story we would just go on because the topic has been sufficiently strip-mined. On the contrary, the topic is encouraged to grow, bidden to remain.

Perhaps this paper is about re-reading and re-membering and how the text(ures) of the earth each read into each

other, so you never have the whole story and you can never
be done with a piece of the story, because it always needs
re-reading into the ongoing generosity of things—the Earth
keeps coming, children keep coming, the task is to keep open
the possibility of re-reading. (Jardine, n.d., p. 7)

Narrative raises questions. Could certain mothers really be extremely worried about testing and we don't realize it? Could we as their care providers be seen as uncaring, even if we care?

The stories can provide a different discussion for novice and expert nurses (Bartol, 1986; Vezeau, 1993; Young-Mason, 1988; Younger, 1990). Novice nurses may not have participated in amniocentesis, for example. Prior to teaching research-based nursing theory about it, I believe it is important to meaningfully bring up the feeling content of the event. By reflecting on the story, novices will likely relate the story to another situation of fear that was more personally experienced. This reflection can help them remain in touch with the significance of the event as they also learn about the theoretical aspects. In this enriched context, we often consider what families might want from nurses before and during such testing activities, beyond the technical information.

For expert nurses, the stories can provide an opportunity to express their own experiences, noting peak events and variances. Expert nurses generally state to me that certain stories permit them, as they look at care situations, to be involved and not distanced, and to be able to express their considerable knowledge about them in very human terms to their students, coworkers, and families. Expert nurses often demonstrate their style of assessment of the emotional needs of families and describe their successes and frustrations in similar care situations.

The difficult work in nursing can lead persons to disengage from their practice; some nurses find it too hard to continue to care. Creative narrative allows practicing nurses to walk around in a singular event, fully involved. By reading the stories, nurses can search for personal meaning, be motivated, and continue to open themselves to the unique circumstances of their patients. Stories can offer a place and a space for needed reflection so that nurses in practice are enabled to provide genuine support, guidance, and a caring presence.

WRITING NARRATIVE

In nursing education and practice, there has been only minimal guidance in the writing of fictional narrative by nurses. While certainly related, the roles of a reader and a writer are entirely different.

Charon (1986) encouraged medical students to write fictionally about patients whom they find are difficult to understand in an environment in which "patients [have] become diseases, and some diseases are more equal than others" (p. 61). Charon's students protect themselves from the sadness and anxiety of their patients by disengagement, but the protection is superficial. In the end, Charon surmises that both students and patients become dehumanized. This dehumanization is specifically what Barry Lopez means by the "failure of imagination"; we can no longer feel ourselves in our own world or see others in it.

Charon helps her students to broaden their own awareness of themselves and their patients by shifting the students' attention to imagine the individual worlds of their patients. In their writing, the students take the perspective of the patients. The writing process shifts the focus of the discomfort by

> . . . *asking for an investment in the texture of that patient's life, and not in the impact of that patient's existence on the student. When one writes, one sees the patient . . . active, living a life. (p. 65)*

The act of writing another's story becomes a dialectic of distance and intimacy through which writers can develop empathy for another and acceptance of their own humanity. The concern is not truth in the sense of "getting it right"; it is the process of honestly projecting oneself into the world of another and seeing it as one's own. Truth here would be the recognition that the nurse and patient inhabit the same world—not in the same way but in the sense of a realization of relation.

There is a concern for nurses who work in multi-cultural set-tings: How are cultures different from their known culture to be represented? The concern in addressing other, alien, cultures (for me, Asian cultures or the situation of stillbirth) is to give the other a story.

My world and that of my patients are not separated by a chasm that neither of us can cross. A nurse who writes fiction does not do so in isolation. As I nurse I live in the context of most of the stories I write. A story is not a product of pure imagination, if there is such a thing, as if something could be made out of noth-ing. Those nurses who write, out of need or requirement, write stories about areas they have some familiarity with—either as na-tive or as stranger. They are not flies on the walls; they are ac-tively engaged with patients, asking questions, and trying not to make assumptions about their lives. If anything, I believe this is what nurses do particularly well—tread in unknown territory and try to determine how foreign or familiar the territory is.

I began thinking about these parallel systems, where, if the two cultures were traveling side by side, you could make in-quiries across the chasm. That's what the shaman does. To my way of thinking, that is also what the scientist does, and the writer in another way. They reach across some danger-ous chasm, where they are at great risk, to inquire of a paral-lel culture, to ponder another order, for how it might illuminate some part of their own culture. (Lopez, in Lued-ers, 1989, p. 17)

In the close intimacy of caring, nurse and patient share individ-ual interpretations of events. Even though I may not thoroughly understand a Latina's context of home, I can listen well. I can be tolerant of my own humanity and provide in my story what I can understand of context, and illuminate what I understand as the meaning content. As I write, I seek advice and confirmation from other women of similar background. It is not exact or certain, but it is an attempt to build the best bridge possible, realizing still that it is very much my own version of a story I am telling, not the chronicle of an event (Bartol, 1986). Bridges do not always hold, but sometimes they do.

Personal Benefits of Writing

Nurses who are encouraged to write may reap considerable benefits. These are unique to each person, but it may be helpful to clarify this idea by describing my own experience.

I have gained special personal benefits from writing. Writing teaches me about who I am. I accept and learn from failure when a story doesn't work. I learn to accept uncertainty in taking a walk when I don't really know where I am going to end up. I can quiet my own internal critics in my writing. I trust that writing is moving me to new areas, toward growth. Writing is an act of kindness toward myself.

Writing takes me very deep under my own veneer, creating a magic in which I can move through the pain of a situation. That is not to say there is always a happy ending. Most often, it is just the opposite. Writing a story helps me not to be caught in a tragedy, but to see the other colors that surround it.

Writing is a way of stepping forward and speaking my voice. It is my most political act. I invite others for their openness to see a familiar situation in a new way. I like to write the usual, the everyday of women's lives, which is often devalued. The everyday is the stuff of our lives. The peaks are not.

I write from reflection, imagination, words, and whatever else preoccupies me along the way. I use the lens that I have developed within my nursing practice. A primary aspect that stands at the fore concerns health. Admittedly, it is usually not in the sense of germs and broken bones, but health in terms of harmony with self and surroundings. In many stories, I write about what a nurse might see in it and the issues she might want to address.

Congruence of Creative Writing and Clinical Practice

My writing is similar to my clinical practice as a nurse. If I do it well, I learn to lose the desire for control over the outcome. I blur usual parameters. In both, I learn to stay in my body in the situation, and not just in my head. I can smell and sense texture. I can feel joy, fear, and uncertainty. I learn to simply hold hands with those for whom I care as well as with my characters. I do this sometimes with my eyes open, and sometimes with my eyes closed and breath held. I learn to trust the perceptions at the edge of my awareness and go where I feel the energy. Expert nurses become experienced in this state of trusting the self and trusting the other so that both get to the other side.

In clinical work as well as writing, I learn to "cut the fat" to try to find the importance which very often is not all peak experiences, but what usually goes unnoticed. Clinical work and writing are similar in that both are full of endless details and little plots. The small events, the little stories, are the important events. In both clinical work and writing, I work to find shape and meaning for streams of experiences.

Admittedly, when I write what I do not know, there is a danger of getting the story wrong, of creating shallow or implausible characters. No inquiry is infallible; all carry risk of failure. I do not think this means I must limit myself to the small repertoire of events that I have personally experienced. The mission in writing fictional narrative, as in all inquiry, is to better understand what one does not know. If the writer knew all there was to an experience, there would not be any need to write it. All writing is exploration into the unknown.

Dialectic of Writing Narrative and Theory

A story is often a reaction to a theory or a general proposition about life. Theory can carry constraints socially and individually even if not intended. A good example is the maternal role theories developed by Rubin (1967) and Mercer (1985). Both are middle-range, predictive theories based in sociology, staging the maturation of women into the mothering role. As such, they are not nursing theories per se, but they represent perhaps the most used theory-based maternal–child nursing programs of education and nursing care. Because they are general statements based on composites, however, they are often limited to inform individual nursing care in clinical practice.

The Rubin and Mercer theories do not take into consideration an individual's past or the present environment. That is not the purpose of theory. Nurses, informed by this theory, have labeled some mothers as inadequate when a mother does not fit the mold. Maternal role theory does summarize the behavior of many women, but it does not address how practitioners might address women who are the exceptions to the theory. Theory has limitations in informing me about individuals. When I walk into a woman's hospital room, I shelve my books of theory where they are in view but not in the way. Theory continues to inform me—I don't disregard the theory—but it remains in the background and cannot replace or overcome the individual patient.

There is broader-range theory that does not take as literal a prescriptive stance toward patients. Watson's theory of human care (1985) is an excellent example. Metaphorically, it is not a book that remains in the background. Watson's theory creates a fame through which unique interaction can be enjoyed between nurse and patient. Watson's theory can help me understand interactions in general, and so helps me brave the unknown. It can not tell what I will find, but perhaps what I should find.

Story does not have the same difficulty in clinical use, however. The purpose of story is different. Its function is not to generalize, but to enlarge the vision of individual possibilities. A story continually adds another outlier, another unique situation, in great detail. Because of this, a story cannot lead to theory.

A story is a way to clarify my ideas and my stance toward theory. A theory provides a watermark that helps me identify who I am. Theory and story are related in a paradigm dialectic. Neither is in opposition; rather, they are intimately related, each helping to define the other.

How to Know Whether We Are Doing It "Right"

This subheading is intentionally tongue-in-cheek. Jardine, who has written extensively on the use of narrative in education, would reply:

[Practice] is thus not a method that can be handed over, but it is practice. It is a practice in a strong sense precisely

> *because the incident under consideration and the concrete*
> *context of speaking about it . . . will have something to*
> *say about what a good interpretation might be in this case*
> *or that. (Jardine, 1992, p. 60)*

After all, narrative can be used in a "this means that" way, as spoken to earlier in this chapter. But this way is not a movement toward enhanced understanding.

> *To teach an understanding . . . is not merely a matter of*
> *putting oneself forward and successfully asserting one's own*
> *point of view, but being transformed into a communion in*
> *which we do not remain what we were. (Gadamer, 1989,*
> *p. 379, quoted in Jardine, 1992, p. 60)*

Movement of the engaged reader is the criterion of "doing it right."

Jardine and Clandinin (1987) described a pedagogical method (of sorts) in "Does It Rain on Vancouver Island?: Teaching as Storytelling." In using a poem by Barry Stevens as a primary metaphor in his text, Jardine suggested that while we may set out to examine the question of rain on Vancouver Island, it is quite peripheral to the educational effort. What emerges may be other, as important, less important, and more important tales. What is critical is that understanding of our world emerges.

> *But storytelling for us in not a matter of the teacher producing an "engaging" story and then implementing it. It is not*
> *a matter of implementation but emergence . . . essentially*
> *dialogical, not monological. (Jardine & Clandinin, 1987,*
> *pp. 477-478)*

In that sense, dialogue would build a community, a family of those linked not only by experiences, but also by the social exchange of read and written experiences, and by peripheral, seemingly tangential shared experiences. This does not come in a "this means that" approach to narrative, but in letting dialogue wander and in our listening to the unsaid.

. . . in the telling of the tales, new members are brought in and these new members transfigure the tales, adding themselves and their flesh to the corpus of the Earth, keeping it going, not essentially/identically, but in kind. (Jardine, n.d., p. 35)

MULTIPLICITY

Nursing has chosen an alliance almost solely with the sciences. In a profession predicated on caring and relationship, this is problematic. If nursing's alliance with science excludes other possibilities or remains in a dominant posture toward the arts and humanities, our inquiry becomes distanced, based on pooled results exterior to us.

All too often . . . educators believe that the sciences have more immediate, if not greater, relevance for nursing. In their opinion, the humanities simply add a fine veneer. . . . Educators who are convinced that nursing has perpetuated a practice-oriented doing culture to the prejudice of its intellectual development welcome the ascendance of science in nursing. . . . Nursing needs a scientific stance but not to the prejudice of art. . . . Knowledge of anatomy and physiology as well as technical skills are essential for nursing, but unless it is tempered with a humanistic orientation, nursing will be less than successful. (Bartol, 1986, p. 21)

My vision for nursing is a conscious alliance among those nurses pursuing science and those pursuing art and humanities. Blending cannot be the goal, because the goals of inquiry are at odds. In slight contrast to Bartol, I want the arts and humanities not simply to temper science, but to be on equal footing. Nursing can strive toward a fuller dialectical relationship, valuing both science and art, because both are needed to inform our understandings of health and transition.

. . . the storyteller has always had this central role in societies of translating information. . . . So the factual

> *information we get and the new metaphors created out of*
> *science somehow have to be translated into the language of*
> *the storyteller—by film, by speech, by literature, by any*
> *means that will make it meaningful and powerful to the hu-*
> *man mind. (Lopez, quoted in Lueders, 1989, p. 26)*

Nowhere is this more needed in nursing than education and practice.

Readers and writers of narrative can help nursing to understand the clinical world of caring, not purely in terms of the general but in the diverse particular. Nursing can value and encourage the storytellers in our community for the products that evoke contact with what was not previously understood, as well the process, the attention to nuances, that makes stories possible.

Narrative will not show the road to take when a comparable situation is met again; it is not prescriptive. Narrative can help nursing see alternatives and be fully engaged in caregiving. Its role is to compel us to hesitate, to question our reflex responses, and to remember the individual exception.

NARRATIVE: AN EXAMPLE

Writing stories helps me to understand experiences. By living in an experience for an extended period of time, I learn to find the words to express it. I remain embodied, smelling the smells and seeing the colors.

As a nurse, I do not cure. I can rarely take away the worst of pain or sorrow, and create happiness in their stead. As a nurse, I am most often an engaged witness, a person who can hold a version of reality in my heart as we all move through profound experiences. Each time it is different—scary, violent, intense, exhilarating, wonderful, and privileged.

For all that has been written about aesthetic knowing, little aesthetic work has been encouraged or published. This volume is a remarkable exception, and I appreciate the opportunity to share an original work of fiction.

Hair, Smells, Spaces

"Mama, please . . . water . . . I am so tired. . . . this will never end. Uh . . . again, oh no, not again . . . Mama!"

This room smelled of many odors. One smell was Señora Peña's flowery bath water from the night before—gardenias whose bouquet only got stronger over time. Her sweat flowed in small rivers between her ample hovering breasts and converged with the wetness of the wide belt around her rayon dress. The cooking odor of cocoa butter remained on the señora's hands from hours ago when she softly massaged her daughter's smallish hips to help the pain, to relax the muscles, to widen the way for this first, big, and resistant baby.

Elena carried "Essence of Birth" on her body and in the musky spaces between her and the bed, and between her and the others in the room. The fluid from inside her had gushed not long ago. There was no time to clean the bed so the nurse had simply put dry blue bed protectors under her. There were too many. They stuck to her skin. They carried their own sharp plastic smell that battled with the waters that broke. Their smell soured and embittered the slightly sweet, sweaty smell of the water that carried the first idea of what her baby would whiff of.

Elena's breath added to the mixture in the small spaces near her face. The breath had a distinctive smell. It was dry and hot, exhausted, flavored with a mint sprig her mother had given her to chew on. Her breath's boundaries ebbed and flowed from Elena, panting close to her face and her pillow. Then Elena's breath would explode with noise, spilling the woman's energy, fear, pain into spaces near the cabinets and near mother and near the other attendants in the room to be smelled and absorbed. In-out, in-out. In-OUT. It depended on what her body was doing at the time. And the baby, too.

The nurse smelled—much to her dismay. She always put deodorant on before coming to work, but it never contained all the aromas of remembered births (her own and all the others), her children, dinner from the night before, her sweat from the radiator hotness of these women at hard labor, her overheated feet, and the aromas of her fear and her hopes for each woman.

There were other people in the room—vague and obligatory and officiating attendants—but, oddly, they gave off little smell. This happens when there is little interest, little engagement, as was the case with these attendants. Luckily, the non-smells simply took a seat in the corner and thumbed through some old magazines and did not get in the way of these three women in the room.

Many of the other smells in the room didn't have a chance. They sulked for a while. (You know: in the corners of the counters where the alcohol wipes live with the bandaids inside their flimsy paper wrappers; the blue gel that laid between the monitor pad and Elena's belly, over the baby's backside; and the oil that kept all the vigilant machines in the room working.) Yes, they were jealous, but they had seen this before. They were overcome by the smells Elena, her mother, and the nurse brought into (made in) this room. Sometimes, birth was simply too much for the usual hospital-room smells to dominate. Well, with the better births anyway. Better ones? Well, those with people in the room—real people who did sweat and cry and give up and go on and give birth and grip hands and lift heavy thighs and sense sad things and happy things and surprising things.

All this makes powerful smells. Even the father standing outside the doorway sent his scent under the curtains that blocked his view. (This was his wish. He was not sure, not certain, even though Elena was. His body means, he thought the baby was his, probably was. He wanted it to be—although he didn't tell her that. But that time last year when he got too big, too strong with her and they parted for a short while until their bodies couldn't stand it any longer. That time away meant he couldn't be sure, couldn't be certain. The baby felt like his own. The baby returned his touch to her belly with a kick every time. He loved her. He loved the baby. But his place was here. It was convenient that it was usual, but it was also that he wasn't sure.)

It is unclear if he meant to do so, exactly—willing his scent to be sent to her. That is, he wanted to be with his wife—and not; but he felt her pain, her moans, her fear, her resignation, and a little happy anticipation. He knew (but did not consciously think this, his body thought this) that no one else in the room could know this part—the part about the little happy anticipation. That's a smell only he knew about Elena. So, he sent some back to her (not his brain, his body wanted to do so). His fear, his tiredness, his pain, his desire, and his little happy hope all floated under the hospital curtains that screened only the visible from others.

Elena, in that world between the pains, whispered, "Xavier."

Elena's wet hair stuck around her lips and in the corners of her mouth. Hair is a great prop for the emotions. Elena normally wore her hair, well, in a way that always was her. Her bangs were dark, dark black (maybe a little brownish if you looked very hard) and rose straight up many inches above her face. Up and then slid down in an ocean's wave toward her left ear. It was a tiara without jewel, but often there was enough hairspray that her hair often sparkled in the evening as the sun set and she was outside talking to girlfriends across from her mother's house. They were a majestic sight to see, these bangs. One doesn't really need to even mention the rest of her hair—it paled in beauty by comparison. It was simply the chorus surrounding the action above her eyes.

But not today. Her hair had special plans for today that would embrace the birth and the hair would step back and encourage the birth's governance of the senses. Elena's hair contained and administered the smells closest, such as Elena's breath, and her mother's breath caressing Elena's ear as her mother held Elena's right leg up and out while Elena pushed, lying on her side. The hair laid loose—wet and stringy on anything it touched. But it did not pull against Elena's head. There was enough pain and struggle in the room. Always, the hair moved with Elena, holding tight to her face, her shoulder and neck, but did not hurt and did not call attention to itself.

Other hair on Elena's body helped the birth. Arm hair rubbed against hips lifting the cocoa butter smell, soothing, closer to Elena's nose as her hands clung to the pillow above her head while she pushed, while her body tried to convince the baby more and more persuasively to come out, to be welcomed, to be held in arms instead of belly.

Private hair, curly and wet, cooled the hothouse heat at the entrance to the baby when Elena's breath gushed out with a scream. It was so hot there, right there—steamy, jungle-ly, mysterious. One could almost see long-leaved ropes of lush green vegetation with the eyes of unseen occupants peering through. It was hot there—wet, vaporous, swollen— and only the occasional breeze of Elena's breath cooled it. And so the hair accepted the soft wind and held it in its wetness, and gave a moment's coolness to Elena and the unseen occupant.

There was a rustle in the immediate hush of the room.

"The head . . . Xav . . . the head . . . it hurts . . . oh, mama, please make him come out . . . mama. . . . "

"All right, Elena, you've really got to push now with the next one, his tones are going down . . . ."

Elena was lost—her body no longer heard or saw anything. Her eyes squeezed shut and her ears, too. Only smell and pain and wetness and hot and baby were in her world now. No mother, no Xavier, no hospital, no room, no bed, no future. Only now and pressure and her body turning itself inside out, pushing the inside out, pushing the pain away from her, pushing the baby (no more pleading and sweet-talk—this was serious now)—now. Elena's body brooked no interruption, accepted no calls, heard no advice, but smelled the mother, smelled the nurse, felt the sharpness and bitterness of wanting/having to let go and the push, the urgency, the head pressing and stuck and not moving, pressing and staying right there.

Without the nurse seeing, the mother rubbed a trifle of cocoa butter from Elena's hips around the side of the baby's head. The baby's head moved against that hand of the mother's and pushed with his feet—stretching toward the hand and the cooking smell and the smell of sweat and old gardenias. The baby became . . . curious.

The rhythm in the room beat the drum harder until all three women were moving as in the same wave, slightly pulled toward Elena's right hip, and then down. Then the nurse like a dolphin that breaks the surface of the wave and dives under for pure joy, rose up and leapt downward with grace and smoothness to the jungle hotness of the curly hair now being cooled by the breath of all three women and plunged down to meet the child, and gave advice to the baby's body—right shoulder, turning the head, left shoulder and backside and feet, and broke surface finally out of breath, panting, blowing, putting baby back to belly but within arms of Elena and her mother.

The baby did not look or hear (eyes and ears squeezed shut) but with his first breath took in the smells of the three women, cocoa butter, gardenias, and remembered births. Then another smell reached his nose from the space between his cord and Elena's soggy belly, and he wrinkled his nose and took in a touch of pain and fear and hope from beyond the women. The smell, his father, moved closer to see his son.

The clean disinfected attendants swarmed out of the corners to focus their eyes and their brains on this infant boy and found—a problem. It really wasn't a problem—it was only a difference—but to them it was a problem. That is, really wasn't a problem—nothing is done—it is common enough—but then—they started to smell. It was a shark smell, a predator smell, a more-than-mild-interest smell. It was a "soon the problem will be for me to explain, and console, and control—that is my job" smell.

One doctor pointed to the small left foot of the baby. It had a sole, a palm, an ankle, bones, and toes—six of them. The father looked, the grandmother looked, but Elena was not in their world yet (she didn't look).

Xavier and the grandmother did not look and they did not hear as the doctor started explaining and justifying and comforting, and the father's and the señora's smells overcame—no, expanded—to fill all the spaces of importance in the room: the space between the baby's left elbow and Elena's left nipple, the infinitely small space between Xavier's left hand pressing into his mother-in-law's hand, all the important spaces. Their smell was more compelling, sweeter, grander, and their smell was that of relief and joy.

Without willing it (but the body willed it), Xavier's left foot worked its way out of its shoe.

"Yes, yes . . . ," Elena's mother whispered softly, blowing great love and affection for this freed young man on her breath into his left ear.

Xavier reached down and removed his left sock, white, clean, smelling softly of love and connection with his son. Xavier's hot, sweaty foot almost resisted the cool, white, clean floor, as Xavier fanned and wiggled his toes in the space above the floor and between his toes. Both father and son wiggled and flexed and fanned their left toes—all twelve of them. Elena, still in her body's world, began to surface to the shared world, and smiled at the smell of recognition so close to her, in her hair.

REFERENCES

Aoki, T. (1991). *Pedagogical storying/theming: Toward practitioners' understanding of teaching through narratives.* Unpublished paper.

Banks, J. (1990). Literature as a clinical capacity: Commentary on "The Quasimodo complex." *The Journal of Clinical Ethics, 1*(3), 227-231.

Bartol, G. (1986). Using the humanities in nursing education. *Nurse Educator, 11*(1), 21-22.

Bartol, G. (1989a). Creative literature: An aid to nursing practice. *Nursing and Health Care, 10*(8), 453-457.

Bartol, G. (1989b). Story in nursing practice. *Nursing and Health Care, 10*(10), 564-565.

Charon, R. (1986). To render the lives of patients. *Literature and Medicine, 5,* 58-74.

Gadamer, H.-G. (1989). *Truth and method.* New York: Crossroad Books.

Gadow, S. (1985). Robots, despots, and cronies. *Humanities and the Health Professions* (No. 8), 17-26.

Gadow, S. (1990a, May). *Beyond dualism: The dialectic of caring and knowing.* Paper presented at a meeting of the International Association for Human Caring, Houston, TX.

Gadow, S. (1990b). Response to "Personal knowing: Evolving research and practice." *Scholarly Inquiry for Nursing Practice, 4*(2). (Preliminary version)

Jardine, D. (1988). Speaking with a boneless tongue. In Bas Leverng (Ed.), *Pedagogy in the postmodern era.* Publisher unknown.

Jardine, D. (1992). "The fecundity of the individual case:" Considerations of the pedagogic heart of interpretive work. *Journal of Philosophy of Education, 26*(1), 51-61.

Jardine, D., & Clandinin, D. (1987). Does it rain on Vancouver Island?: Teaching as storytelling. *Curriculum Inquiry, 17*(4), 471-481.

Lopez, B. (1989). *Arctic dreams: Imagination and desire in a northern landscape.* New York: Bantam Books.

Lueders, E. (1989). *Writing natural history: Dialogue with authors.* Salt Lake City: University of Utah Press.

Mercer, R. (1985). The process of maternal role attainment over the first year. *Nursing Research, 34*(4), 198-203.

Parker, R. S. (1990). Nurses' stories: The search for a relational ethic of care. *Advances in Nursing Science, 13*(1), 31-40.

Rubin, R. (1967). Attainment of the maternal role: Part I, Processes. *Nursing Research, 6*(2), 230-237.

Stone, J. (1985). Medicine and the arts. *Theoretical Medicine, 6*(10). (Preliminary version)

Vezeau, T. (1993). Storytelling: A practitioner's tool. *Maternal Child Nursing, 18*(4), 193-196.

Vitz, P. (1990). The use of stories in moral development: New psychological reasons for an old education method. *American Psychologist, 45*(6), 709-720.

Watson, J. (1985). *Nursing: Human science and human care.* Norwalk, CT: Appleton-Century-Crofts.

Webster, G. (1990). Nursing and the philosophy of science. In J. McCloskey & H. Grace (Eds.), *Current issues in nursing* (3rd ed.). St. Louis: Mosby.

Woolf, V. (1929). *Women and writing.* New York: Harcourt.

Younger, J. (1990). Literary works as a mode of knowing. *Image: The Journal of Nursing Scholarship, 22*(1), 39–43.

Young-Mason, J. (1988). Literature as a mirror to compassion. *Journal of Professional Nursing, 4*(4), 299–301.

Part III

Art as Practice

9

The Art of Painting
Meets the Art of Nursing

Karen Breunig

*T*his chapter is about the connection between the art process and the art of nursing. I am a painter and a nurse. I try to be an artist at both. Ten years ago I could not have conceived of their connection. Today, I know the challenge of living that connection. My journey to this place has been both rich and frightening. Let me set the scene.

Twenty years ago, I became a nurse. My mother, a practical Irish woman, gave her daughters two choices: teacher or nurse. I chose the latter. Hospitals had always drawn me with their promise of the drama of birth and death. I wanted to be there where the mystery of entering and exiting took place. The humanness of it all seduced me.

My father, a little less practical, a dreamy kind of man, taught us about art and the world's great painters. In his little workshop behind the garage, he was an alchemist with oil paint. I saw him turn red to purple before my eyes. And I saw sunlight pour from the end of a brush across a landscape of his making. There was something outside of ordinary humanness about it. It too seduced me and still does.

Art school was out of the question for this daughter of a practical Irish woman. So I finished nursing school in four years, worked as a pediatric nurse for three years, and saved every spare cent to pay for art school tuition. I eventually enrolled in graduate school in painting in Manhattan, the center of the universe for artists at that time. To pay the bills, I worked in a nursing home on the weekends, grateful that I had a "practical" skill to fuel this not-so-practical passion. That was about the only connection between nursing and art that I was conscious of. And there I stayed for more than 10 years.

At one point, I left nursing to work part-time running my husband's business. The remainder of the week I spent inside my studio, traveling to the ends of my interior world and back. Over and over again, year in and year out, I came back to the same images, the same obstacles, the same challenges, the same fears, and I came to know them on an intimate basis. The process of painting became a discipline and a practice. It took on a rhythm and life of its own, and it became as important as the final product had ever been.

It would happen again and again, without any warning. I would work anxiously and laboriously for days, even months. I would come to the near end of my tolerance. I would furiously try to control all aspects of a painting until they became like a million loose threads on a loom that was hell-bent on weaving itself. Then something very subtle would shift in me. I would give up trying to hold on to the reins. It would flow through me, as if I were an open conduit. There would be timeless time. When I looked up some moments or hours later, there would be an image on the canvas that was not of my own doing. There was a rightness about the forms and colors before my eyes. They were exactly as they needed to be. I would feel changed by that image and that experience. It was outside of ordinary humanness. It kept me coming back again and again to the anxiety of the blank canvas.

I built a respectable career as an artist. An old, established New York gallery took me into its stable of artists and gave me a solo show. I began to sell paintings. I began also to forget about nursing, to forget that I had ever been so seduced by the human drama that nurses partake in every day.

The day came when my marriage ended and all life as I had known it was called into question. I was forced by circumstance to turn again to the nursing I thought I had left far behind. My art career alone could not support my daughter and myself. I had to reconcile that part of myself I had seen as "practical" with those parts of myself I knew as creative. I had no idea where this reconciliation would lead. I only knew I was frightened.

The creative process I had known for years in the studio, was beginning to eek its way out of my studio door and into my "outside" life. It is something I had yearned to understand and feel, how one could live one's life outside the studio, experiencing these extraordinary moments in your everyday life. Truly, I thought, one would find a deep passion for living if one could somehow bring those creative moments out into the world.

My work as a nurse had always involved children. So had my work as an artist. I taught art to children in my studio in the summers and had met a group of children from a therapeutic foster home. Each of them was under psychiatric care. They came to my studio to play and explore. They taught me a lot. Again, I was seduced by the drama of life and death, by the drama of their lives. How could I be with these children in ways that would be helpful to them and would be creative?

I have always believed in children's creativity as a source of health. I believe that for my own creativity too. But what does being creative have to do with being a nurse? In the hope that graduate school would answer that question for me, I enrolled.

This is what I have come to understand since that time.

When Watson (1988) wrote about the transpersonal caring relationship and the actual caring occasion, she was writing about the creative moment. In the creative moment of an artist, there is a person, paint, and canvas. In the caring moment, there is a nurse, a client, and the circumstances of their lives. The tools are not brush and canvas; they are empathy, reflection, metaphor, reframing, and caring. The moment when "It," as the Zen master would call it, moves through me feels the same to me in the studio as it now does with a client. These are those timeless times when all comes together and comes through me, when the right thing happens at the right moment, and I am left with no doubt about the rightness and the presence of something outside of ordinary humanness that has revealed itself. I think this is what Heidegger calls "aletheia" or "unconcealment." He has said that art reveals to us not knowledge about any thing but the highest form of knowledge, knowledge of the truth (cited in Sebba & Boers, 1987). It is this truth that I yearn for. Painting is one way of experiencing it. Caring is another. I think this is what Jean Watson was talking about.

What seduction these creative times hold! I will come back again and again. It makes no matter to me if they manifest as color and form on a canvas or new color and form in a relationship. I will remember the otherworldliness of them and it will give me the strength to push through the inevitable creative anxiety—the anxiety that always seems to be there. After all, where there is creation there is destruction. I feel it right now as I write these words. I am up against the anxiety of letting go of my old self, of letting that self die, the self who thought she could not have written these words, who could not possibly have been so competent, who would never have challenged her mother's dictum to be practical and not creative. There will always be a death where there is a birth. There will always be the anxiety of the unknown. We will not know who we will be until we get there.

So goes the process for our clients. We stand alongside them, called on to be the midwives of creativity. We have the honor of being beckoned into their worlds at a time of upheaval and change. There will undoubtedly be great anxiety. What or who is it that is about to be born? What new form will be created in their lives? How is it that we will partake of the moment when "It" flows? We wait with them at the threshold. We wait at the point of highest tension.

When I was deep in the midst of my first small understanding of the creative process in my painting, I read a wonderful little book called *Zen in the Art of Archery,* by Eugen Herrigel (1981). He was a German philosophy professor who, in the 1930s or 1940s, went

to Japan to teach. In an effort to better understand the Eastern
mind, he enrolled as a student of a Zen archery master. For a few
years, the master concentrated his instruction on one skill alone:
drawing the bow properly. The philosophy professor stood alongside the other students, day in and day out, with his bow drawn,
awaiting the word from the master that he could progress to shoot-
ing the arrow. His Western mind grew impatient. How could so
much time be wasted on one seemingly unimportant piece?
Surely, he felt, hitting the target was the most important skill of
all. Many months went by and he looked to his master for some
indication of when the next step would be taken. Finally, the master felt they were ready. He told them only this: They must draw
their bow and wait, without purpose, at the point of highest tension. There they must wait until "It" moves through them and
shoots the arrow.

The years spent perfecting the skill of drawing the bow make
me think about the place of technical skill and discipline in the
practice of a craft and about the marriage of craft with art. I think
the Zen master has much to teach nurses about what the art of
nursing is and how it is wedded to the craft of nursing.

I was in art school in the late 1970s, the end of the hippie era
when we were all being encouraged to "go with the flow" and "do
our own thing." Many art programs in universities were also
"going with the flow." Students were being encouraged to express
themselves on canvas, yet nowhere were we being taught the technical skills of drawing, form, color, or even stretching canvases. It
was all being called art. I was secretly horrified. A lot of it looked
like self-pretentious schlock to me, but I kept my mouth shut for
fear of seeming "old-fashioned." I found a more traditional graduate school, where art was taught in what was called the "atelier"
method. This method harked back to the times when young art
students learned the concrete skills of the craft of painting in the
studios (ateliers) of masters. In my program, we learned how to
mix color and how to stretch and prime a canvas. We were given
the formulas for the painting mediums of the renaissance masters.

We drew and drew and drew, day in and day out. We went to a
museum and stood in front of the world's great paintings and listened, enraptured, to a most passionate man tell of his love affair

with these works. We copied these works in charcoal and in paint, hoping that their great mysteries would thereby be revealed to us. And hoping too that they would teach us the more basic skills of composition, color, and form. They proved to be fine teachers. For every great artist of human remembrance was, first of all, a great craftsman. They all served an apprenticeship. They all spent time learning to "draw the bow" properly. Then, at some point, they were ready to let "It" flow through them, to be an artist. If the bow isn't drawn properly, "It" finds no avenue through which to flow. This I have learned from my own experience.

To become a fine craftsman is no small feat. To become a fine, competent, technical nurse in today's very technical world is no small feat either. Trying to be an artist before one is a fine craftsman is placing the cart before the horse. During my first days as a nursing student, I found myself with a patient in pain. All I prayed for was the skill to administer an injection of pain medication without increasing my patient's discomfort with a sloppy technique. If you had tried to tell me about the art of nursing at that moment, I wouldn't have heard a word. But I would have wanted to know anything you could have told me about the technical skills I needed to be a competent nurse.

Toward the end of my nursing education, I had the great fortune to have a clinical instructor who was both a skilled craftsman and great artist. I remember starting to have the glimmer of understanding that she was different from a lot of the technically good nurses I had watched practice in my clinical placements. Her parting words to me as she handed me my evaluation have come back to me. She told me that she felt I would go on to contribute something of great creativity to my profession. I stared at her blankly. What on earth was she talking about? Was I going to go on to invent a new colostomy bag? I left that rotation perplexed but still moved by her words. I had never heard anyone link creativity to anything but concrete activities with concrete products as their outcomes, like paintings or colostomy bags—objects we could all see.

Now, I think I understand, and Jean Watson is no small part of that understanding. The big creativity, the creativity that permeates one's life, that seeps out of artists' studios and into their lives, expresses itself in creative moments and caring moments alike. Sometimes there is a product to look at and touch; sometimes there is not. The creative product may be a new way of seeing, a new way of approaching one's life and challenges. Sometimes it is a more authentic way of living—or of dying. In a caring moment, we nurses get to participate in the creative process with our clients, and it is genuine caring that plugs us into it. The Zen master might call it "cultivating right mind." Authentic caring is what turns the nurse craftsman into the nurse artist. That is what Jean Watson writes about.

At the end of my art education, I was told by a wise mentor and teacher, "Now go back to your studio and forget everything we ever taught you, and just paint like your life depended on it." That's how he told me to become an artist. I think he was telling me to let my skills become unconscious and to care like I had never cared before. When skills become second nature and we can forget about them on a conscious level, we can move on to the artistry in our practice. Now that I understand that, I understand my apprenticeship as a nurse craftsman and I see the possibility of practicing nursing as an art. To do that, we need to care like we've never cared before, maybe to care like our lives depend on it.

Caring is not easy. It is not Hallmark cards with kind words. It is not a self-indulgent throwing of paint on a canvas. It is a disciplined practice. Often it is damned hard. It demands bringing the authentic self to the caring moment or not showing up at all. My authentic self is not always readily available. She sometimes lies buried under mounds of anxiety. There have been many times when I was there without her, just as there have been many times when I have approached a blank canvas with a mind full of expectations, inadequacies, fears, and the need to control the outcome. I remember struggling at those times but I don't ever remember being creative. Yet I was able to come back to that struggle over and over again because I had the memory of times past when there was timeless time and rightness about the moment. Those times fuel my courage. It takes courage to create and it takes courage to care. You never know who you will be once you've really cared.

Recently, I finished an internship at a community mental health center. I worked on the child, adolescent, and family services team. I worked as an individual therapist and I had ample opportunity to experience caring and creative moments. To some of them I brought my authentic self, to others I brought my cluttered, anxious mind. For almost three years, I have been taught the technical skills of the nurse psychotherapist by some skilled craftsmen and master artists. When I walked into the room to encounter my first client, it was my technical skills I worried about. Could I establish rapport, could I pace and lead, could I pick up on the family dynamics that were being played out under my nose? Then, at some point, I began to care more about the nervous 13-year-old boy in front of me than I cared about being the perfect therapist. I let all the skills I had gathered move down into my cells and become a part of me. Then I could forget about them and know they would make themselves available at just the right moments. I could then be with this boy as my authentic self. That's when artistry becomes a possibility.

I think back to my work in the pediatric ICU and I wonder about the artistic possibilities such places hold. They are the domain of many great nurse craftsmen. I think of these nurses as technical wizards. Technical wizardry is of life-and-death importance in ICUs. There are so many skills to incorporate, so many to make second nature. Skills matter a great deal there. A nurse could spend years just learning to "draw the bow" properly. Perhaps it is harder to be an artist where there is so much to know. But maybe the skills themselves are the avenue to artistry. To the Zen master, how long his pupils took to learn to draw the bow did not matter. The practiced discipline of the learning was important, and this process slowly, over time, changed his pupils in subtle ways. It was the cultivation of "right mind." It think of it as cultivation of the authentic self.

When I approach a blank canvas, I am filled with anxiety. It is the creative anxiety I have spoken about, the fear of letting go of the old self. My mind is full of expectations and the need to control the outcome. Over the years, I have developed my own ritual for getting by the anxiety. I sit at my palette table with my back to the empty canvas and I quietly mix colors. I mix whatever colors call to me that day. The focus of my attention is narrowed down to the plastic cup in my hand and the transformations that are going

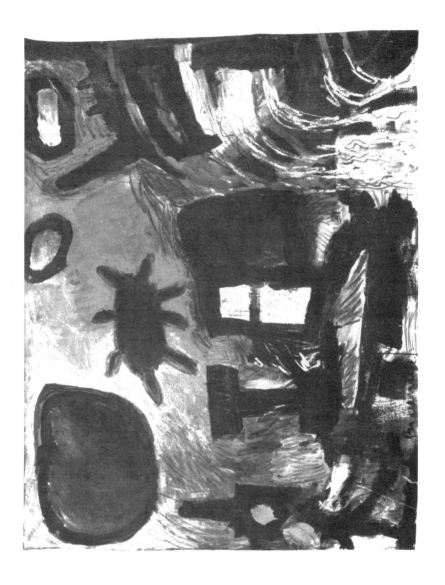

on within its boundaries. After some minutes, I find myself in a trancelike state. Meanwhile, the anxiety and I are coexisting in the same space. I am paying it its due respect. When I don't run from it, I find I can let it be. The trance gets by my defenses, which I think, stand between my authentic self and the canvas. This skill, the mixing of colors, becomes the vehicle for the transcendence of the anxiety and of the craft. It paves the way to artistry. I wonder how this might work in nursing.

The artist in the studio works alone with the empty canvas, the anxiety, and the unconscious process. The nurse works, not alone, but with another human. She brings to the moment her own anxieties, her pain, and her unconscious process. There they intersect with the pain, the anxieties, and the unconscious of the patient. How does she manage all these variables and move them toward a caring moment? What are her tools for unearthing her authentic self? My experience in the studio tells me that if she learns to co-exist with her pain and anxieties, to pay them the respect they are due, her authentic self will find some breathing room. After all the fears and anxieties have made themselves heard and taken a step backward, this self is the one that emerges. With this self, we connect with the pain, anxiety, and unconscious process of our clients. This self is the wellspring of empathy and caring.

Skills can be used to "cultivate right mind," to allow the nurse to coexist in the present moment with her own anxiety and pain, to wait in that moment for them to take their place at the back of her mind and give her authentic self some room to stretch. Does the mindful performing of a second-nature skill put us in a trance that bypasses our defenses? Or do we draw from our sense of competency in the performance of the skill, and from our sense of comfort in the familiarity of the craft, and gain the courage to live with our own pain and anxiety while we open up to our patients'? I am not sure, but I believe that the skills of the painter build the road on which the artist journeys to her authentic self. The skills of the nurse craftsman can do the same.

ICUs are full of opportunities to practice skills again and again. They are full of opportunities to cultivate the authentic self. When a nurse brings herself into the present moment to perform a skilled intervention with a patient, she is walking right into an opportunity to be her authentic self. The skill itself is a tool, like the artist's brush. With her skill, she paints her way right into a caring moment with another human being, and there it is! She has the opportunity to be an artist, to feel something outside of ordinary humanness flow through her, to feel timeless time, to feel that everything about that moment is just as it should be. There are the healing moments, the soul-healing moments. As nurses, we get to share these moments with our fellow humans.

What an honor it is to be a nurse. What an honor it is to be an artist. Even if the caring and creative moments happen only once in a great while, I will forever be seduced by them. They give me the strength to practice the drawing of the bow and the waiting, without purpose, at the point of highest tension.

REFERENCES

Herrigel, E. (1981). *Zen in the art of archery.* New York: Vintage Books.
Sebba, H., & Boers, H. (Eds.). (1987). *Creativity lectures by Gregor Sebba.* Atlanta, GA: Scholars Press.
Watson, J. (1988). *Nursing: Human science and human care.* New York: National League for Nursing.

10

The Power of Creativity in Healing: A Practice Model Demonstrating the Links between the Creative Arts and the Art of Nursing

Mary T. Rockwood Lane
with John Graham-Pole

*T*his chapter describes the evolution of an arts program created against the background of a traditional health care setting. As a nurse and an artist, I have created and founded an Artists in Residence Program. My overall mission is to explore and develop links between the creative arts and healing arts. I have included here my personal story of reclaiming my own artist. In discussion of creativity and practice, the model of the human being is presented and described in metaphorical language. The operationalization and objectives of the Artists in Residence Program are reviewed, and the exact types of art activities included in the arts program are presented. The artist's perspective is shared. The purpose of this chapter is to inspire nursing leadership and implementation in this endeavor.

THE POWER OF CREATIVITY IN HEALING: THE PRACTICE MODEL

The effect in sickness of beautiful objects, of variety of objects and especially of brilliancy of color is hardly at all appreciated. I have seen in fevers (and felt, when I was a fever patient myself) the most acute suffering produced from the patient not being able to see out of window and the knots in the wood being the only view. I shall never forget the rapture of fever patients over a bunch of bright colored flowers. People say the effect is only on the mind. It is no such thing. The effect is on the body, too. Little as we know about the way in which we are affected by form, by color and light, we do know . . . they have an actual physical effect. Variety of form and brilliancy of color in the objects presented to patients are actual means of recovery. (Florence Nightingale, 1888)

The Lady of the Lamp beckons us to the light. We have embarked on a renewed journey of exploring and discovering the possibilities of creativity and healing.

The authors have cocreated an art program within a traditional health care setting. This is happening at Shands Hospital, in Gainesville, Florida, with extraordinary momentum and commitment. Doors have opened and integration of the arts has been invited in. As a nurse and painter, I am committed to creating a practice model that will implement traditional creative art activities in nursing practice.

The overall mission in creating this arts program is to explore and demonstrate links between the creative arts and the healing arts. We see these links as enhancing and integrating our physical, mental, emotional, and spiritual well-being. This program creates new links: artists to patients; nurses to artists; health care administrators, families, art educators, and the many health care disciplines to each other. We have a common goal, and each discipline has a unique perspective on the process of integration.

This chapter describes how artists have been integrated into the patients' care and how nurses have expanded their clinical practice to include the arts. In the evolving partnership, nurses have provided leadership and a genuine commitment to integrate the arts. The practice model described here is based on the foundation of nursing advocacy in the context of the human caring praxis (Watson, 1988), utilizing art as a therapeutic tool. Nursing's unique relationship with patients allows incorporating the arts into care. The purpose of the model is to embrace nursing's nature of advocacy as described by Gadow in her work on clinical subjectivity. Advocacy typically has been understood as assistance to patients in giving voice to their values (Gadow, 1980). The nurse as an art advocate or liaison to the artist is assisting the patient's voice and artistic expression.

The nurse facilitates the patients' creative/artistic expression in the context of caring, for the purpose of enhancing the patient's autonomy and self-determination. In this nurse–patient interaction, the focus is to embrace and allow for the many forms of creative expression. Watson's theory of human caring is the foundational philosophical framework to describe praxis and how the arts are a vital part of our nursing practice. As nurse–artist coordinator and founder of an Artists in Residence Program, I am creating the practice model for the arts to be incorporated into nursing care. Nurses act as liaisons, linking patients with artists, and they advocate each patient's creative process in whatever form the patient is familiar with and/or has interest. Nurses are also exploring possibilities of the role of artist themselves and are bringing their own artistic talents into their practice to enrich their clinical experience. The program encourages us and reminds us: Everyone is an artist.

The basic tenet of this effort is: We believe that we are all artists and that expressing ourselves through art empowers us. When we are ill, we feel helpless, out of control, and uncreative. Art and play restore us. Art is not a specialty available only to "the artist." It is important to reclaim that we are all artists.

Reclaiming My Own Artist

My voice emerged from my personal experience in using art as a vehicle for my own "healing," recovery, and discovery in an illness experience. I lived art as a healing process. I remember the moment of my empowerment as an artist: I was in the painting process and becoming my own healer. This discovery and exploration renewed my spirit, which in turn, enhanced and facilitated my recovery. This occurred several years ago. I was extremely ill, my resources collapsed, and I felt like I was drowning. I was not able to constructively deal with my own life events. Yet, in a lucid moment, I decided to abandon my fears of being a painter—something I had always dreamed of being and had never given myself permission to do because I never felt "good enough." What was good enough? I felt devastated, and the fear of inadequacy was minute compared to what I perceived as a much greater and painful loss.

I created a studio space for myself and simply started to paint. I painted feverishly. At first, I made no attempt to define myself or my process. I painted from a pure feeling state. I was absorbed by expression, gesture, and the release of my energy on the canvas. I began what turned out to be a series of self-portraits. The first painting was called "Cut Out My Heart" (Figure 1). It was pain, deeply intense—a dying pain. The figure was broken, distorted, diffuse, crumpled, crying, and bleeding. I painted "her." This figure was my despair, my uncensored and purely emotional energy. In the moment of releasing this image, I stepped back and looked. What I saw was an aspect of myself I couldn't face; it was too ugly. Yet I felt calm and detached. I was letting go on a powerfully intense emotional and physical level. I backed away, left the studio, and went home. When I returned and saw that the image had captured and contained a moment that was now past, I had an incred-

Figure 1. Oil Painting, "Cut Out My Heart"
(first painting in a series of six self-portraits)

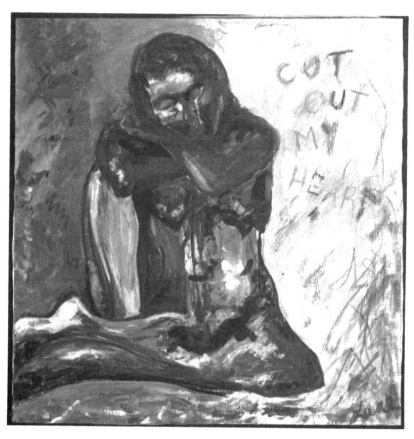

ible insight. The painting remained an object that now contained an image created in genuine and immediately felt expression, and I had moved past it. I realized that movement was occurring. I was witnessing my own transformation.

As I painted this series of self-portraits, I struggled in each painting, with form and perspective. Metaphorically, I was recreating and reconstructing my inner form and inner perspective. The external creative process mirrored my inner world. I realized the power of the manifestation of movement and change: it was a process of knowing myself. As I immersed myself in the painting,

I became not only well but also the artist I always wanted to be—a part of myself I had not acknowledged or honored. From this personal experience, I became confident that art can be used as a vehicle for healing.

My creative process, painting, reflected my inner experience of healing in a particular series of self-portraits. My relationship to these self-portraits has created an awareness and a transformational process in my own life. Art was a way to know myself and the experience of my pain. Seeing it, I could step away—yet it remained an object in the physical world and I became the artist. I validated this lived experience in a constructive way.

THE MODEL OF CREATIVITY IN PRACTICE

My intention was to create a program based on interactive process in which nurses could begin to incorporate the arts as therapeutic activities as well as facilitate a variety of creative activities for themselves and their patients. This approach is based on the philosophy of transcendence, which is deeply rooted in the personal lived experience. As an individual creates art in some form, the artist (i.e., "self") is actualized and the art speaks from within. The wisdom of the body is seen, heard, and felt; it becomes known. In this knowing, facilitated through a creative process, we can confront or simply become aware of ourselves. In our acceptance of and compassion for ourselves, we move on to heal the spirit and the body in terms of loving ourselves clearly, honestly, and compassionately. I believe art reflects an inner reality that gives rise to meanings and offers an opportunity to move forward to a new and expanded consciousness.

We search for wisdom and knowledge, and the focus is knowledge of the self. We assume that everyone is an artist. This "artist" expresses an inner reality that is *meaningful* and authentic. The insight released by this experience is healing. The art form, as it is expressed, becomes part of the external world and there is an opportunity for recognizing the "self" as it is reflected in the art form: To know oneself is to understand oneself. The art form is a way to allow the self to express, release, and discharge energy, thus allowing for acceptance and space for internal healing of the body, mind, and spirit.

I realize I am on a journey of *unfolding* in my own life. I am exploring my own reality and experiencing life as a creative process. This is clear in nature as flowers bloom, the seasons change, babies are born, and death and rebirth are constantly around us. Creativity is the pulsating energy of the universe and the pulsating energy of life. There are infinite possibilities for our creative expression. Our creative work and consciousness open up the experience of living. In whatever form it takes, this is the process of healing. It is being in the world as an open space where our "beingness" comes out of concealment (from ourselves as well as from others) into truth and withdraws again into obscurity (Heidegger, 1977). It is brought to the light for self-interpretation, self-discovery, and self-confirmation.

In exploring the links between the phenomenon of creativity and its power in healing, I am developing a conceptual framework of creativity by explaining and defining how it expands nursing practice. This analysis is a method of organizing practice and examining the attributes of the creative process. My intent is to create a model that will contribute to the scientific knowledge and development of nursing theory. This model must provide the assumptions and guiding principles to implement (1) an art program that expands nursing practice to embrace the use of creative arts as a therapeutic tool and (2) a clinical program that generates knowledge and research based on the clinical experience of how we interface with the arts.

Watson (1993) advocated the nurse as artist, encouraging us to expand the praxis of human caring. The partnership with the artist is appropriate because it offers us another way of seeing and another way of being with our patients. The nurse as artist can bring out the inherent beauty common and integral in our care. We can see the moment as it occurs. We can recognize the beauty that is already present. It is a way of seeing and of being present. It is caring praxis.

Each of us is now being drawn, in one way or another, toward a great vision. It is more than a vision. It is an

*emerging force. It is the next step in our evolutionary jour-
ney. (Zukav, 1989)*

The development of an arts program is itself a creative process
requiring imagination, ingenuity, interest, and personal commitment. It is a process of creative exploration and implementation.
In our vision, the creative arts and the art of nursing will be recognized as being of equal significance as medical and nursing technology continue to progress. The commitment to explore these
links emerged from clinical practice and from my own personal
experience of an illness, when I used painting as a healing process
of personal transformation.

A unique sensitivity of nurses is grounded in the context of
the caring praxis (Watson, 1988). This sensitivity and the nurse's
unique and immediate relationship with the patient and the family
qualify the nurse to introduce the benefits of the arts. Nurses move
in and out of the patients' environment, contribute to creating the
environment, and potentially focus the patients' attention on tasks
to be done and on appreciation of the possible art forms and expressions of beauty that already occur. There is an inherent opportunity to look at the situation differently, validate the gentle wisps
of creative possibilities, and then empower them. Art is about caring. It can be seen as an integral part of how we care, and it embraces the beauty of the moment and our humanness. The nurse
can make visible the invisible, listen to the unsung song or the un-
told story, by simply being there to touch, to hold a hand, to listen
to and encourage the spirit as it strengthens and sings. We can
honor this moment. Our work is in the "art of caring," and art is
caring manifested in a form, a story, a song, a picture, or a dance.
We are the leaders in bringing the arts to fruition in this setting. We
bring together Sister Art with Brother Science, the feminine with
the masculine, love with the facts, nursing with medicine.

Another important assumption is that we are drawing on the
artist within (Edwards, 1986). Healing is understood as the expanding consciousness and the play of the imagination. Healing requires a medium—a form of expression that can serve as a bridge
from the self into the environment. Newman described health as
expanding consciousness. The creative arts serve a therapeutic

role. We accept and facilitate this process, without judgment, in whatever form it takes. We embrace the uniqueness of another and honor the human spirit. The primary function of artistic expression is the joy experienced in the process. The flow in consciousness occurs effortlessly and creates a state of total ease (Csikszentmihalyi, 1990). Art creates movement, patterns are manifest, and there is a release that eases the spirit. The self has a voice. Listening and seeing are part of the healing process.

THE MODEL OF THE HUMAN BEING

My model is constructed to conceptualize the person—the patient, the nurse, the artist—actually any human being—in the process of creativity. The model, shown in Figure 2, presents constructs of import to describe the person and the creative phenomenon. Its

Figure 2. Conceptual Model

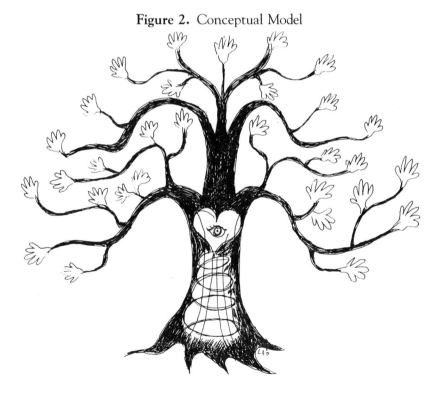

presentation is purely metaphorical. The tree figure (Earth) embraces the "beingness" of the self. The self can be described in relationship with another person in the process of sharing an artistic interaction.

Beingness is central to the self. At the center of the self is a heart, which represents the individual, grounded in the environment and embraced by the earth, and the earth's connection and relationship to the world. The earth perspective is critical. Within the heart is an open eye, representing awareness. Beingness is the life force (spirit and energy) spiraling in a rhythmic pattern of expansion and contraction along the life process. (An ancient symbol for this energy is the snake.) Openness and interconnectedness flow to all aspects of the environment. Creative energy pulsates in the world. The time frame is now—the beingness is in the present; yet in that instant exists all of eternity.

The Self

For the self, the physical form of beingness, I have chosen the symbol of a clear heart. The self is the body (its physical experience and biological functioning), the mind and its thoughts, the emotions and sensations. Humans have the ability to sense the world through perceptual experience—responses of joy, sadness, pain, anger. The heart, at its best, is clear and open. It communicates its beingness into the environment and symbolizes the centeredness of the physical form.

The Eye

The awareness of the self is symbolized by an open eye—seeing oneself being in the world. Being awake implies consciousness and recognition of patterning, of having a mind and body, of having emotions and sensing oneself as a witness to one's own life. The eye is witness to being with life and in the world.

The Hands

The hands represent the movement of creative energy into the environment. Like leaves on a tree, the hands become part of the environment with and of the human being. The hands symbolize the possible empirical referents to be validated by artistic expressions—the physical manifestations of the self, as expressed by the heart with the open eye, which is conscious of the process. Each hand may represent a story, a poem, a drawing or painting, a dance, or even nursing care. Each is a creative art reflecting the self from which it emerged and mirroring a higher level of consciousness back to its creator.

The Tree

The environment is symbolized by a tree that is grounded in and part of the earth. This environment includes physical space as well as family, friends, health care providers, and all external forms. Heidegger (1926) explored in his essays the pursuit of understanding reality by knowing the "thingness" grounded in the context of the earth. The individual, as a participant in the world, is connected to the changing seasons and the groundedness of earth. The earth is celebrated for the protection and nourishment it affords. Heidegger (1926) described individuals' participation in the creative strife of world and earth: they reveal beings and let them come to radiant appearance, allowing all things the darkness and growing time they require to emerge splendidly when they come to the light. These descriptions facilitate an understanding of how art emerges from the darkness within the self into the light of the physical world's acknowledgement.

OPERATIONALIZATION OF THE MODEL

The primary operationalization of my model has been an initial art program in the Bone Marrow Transplant Unit at Shands Teaching Hospital, in Gainesville, Florida. The program's objective is to use art as a therapeutic modality to explore the reality of art and its significance in patient care and in nursing practice.

The position of the nurse is significant. A person with understanding does not know and judge as one standing unaffected but as one united with the other through a specific bond (Gadamer,

1975). This process describes a connection between the nurse and patient as part of a transformation process that is grounded in the earth; energies merge and create something new. Creativity allures us to its infinite possibilities. As a nurse, artist, and researcher, I am committed to a destiny that calls, "Follow your bliss," in whatever form this comes to light for myself, for nursing, and for humanity.

THE ARTISTS IN RESIDENCE PROGRAM

A specific art program has been initiated on the Bone Marrow Transplant Unit and is gradually spreading to other units at Shands Hospital. The primary intent has been to create a program that integrates diverse and multifaceted art activities with the daily routines of patients and their families while providing artistic opportunities for nurses and other health care professionals to share in the process, explore their own creativity, and see themselves as artists.

A performing arts series was initially created to bring the arts to a wider audience all at once. The local Junior League coordinates this activity with the performers and transports patients and families to performances. A strolling artcart brings art supplies to hospitalized children. A Fine Arts Poster Cart will soon allow patients to choose works of art to hand in their hospital rooms. At patient art exhibitions and community art fairs, artists have specifically dealt with the healing process in their artistic work and creative style.

As founder of the Artists in Residence Program, I have worked closely with nurses who see themselves as advocates of the arts in the practice and with artists who are currently implementing the art activities as therapeutic modalities. Initially, our focus was to introduce the creative arts to staff. Among several ongoing workshops are: "Writing for Healing" and "Dancing for the Health of It!" The workshops are open to all health care providers.

Both the nurses and the artists are using their particular medium for individual self-exploration and self-expression. A series of workshops is available to the staff directly on the units. Each artist conducts a workshop to introduce the art materials and activities that are planned for patients and their families. For example, our first artist in residence, at the first unit workshop, used fimo clay to create beads, sculptures, and ornaments for the holidays. Nurses and family members were engaged together on this project. The second workshop offered mixed media and collaborative art projects. Art bins were stocked with supplies and journals, and participants explored ways to create visual diaries and engage in creative writing. Our second artist in residence, a fabric artist, has conducted several T-shirt and hat painting workshops. The initial focus was to get the nurses' feedback and input and then to plan implementation with patients and their families.

Presently, on an oncology unit, we are creating a music program. The artist/musician is conducting programs for the staff and compiling listening libraries that are available to staff and patients. A dancer is now interested in working with movement in the hospital environment, to explore the possibilities of working with children. Tremendous interest has come from artists who appreciate and are interested in the opportunity to expand their creative work into the health care setting. Most artists are volunteers; we provide a small honorarium for their time and supplies. Some nurses who are also writers, musicians, and dancers have been bold and courageous enough to bring their artistic talents into practice. They feel that, in the context of the program, they have permission to be freer and more creative than they are in daily interactions. To communicate the joy in this sharing and caring for each other, it has been extremely important to focus on creating for the nurses an experience in which they can know this process for themselves. A felt lived experience is stronger than words. From a perspective within themselves comes the ability to integrate the arts with confidence, useful application, and fun!

The objectives of the Artists in Residence program are:

1. Use art as a therapeutic modality.
2. Implement an Artists in Residence Program in which the artist facilitates the creative process with the multidisciplinary team.

3. Implement the use of creative art methods and materials with patients, families, and staff.
4. Facilitate art exhibitions in the hospital environment (on the units as well as in common areas) and in the community.
5. Facilitate the development of related art programs and community involvement (music, drama, performing arts, journal-writing groups, and roaming artcarts).
6. Collaborate with the team for development of research protocols using quantitative as well as qualitative methods.

The program has created a partnership with all the health care providers and has established a coordinating and investigative team. Our initial inservice orientation for staff and faculty explains the goals of the Artists in Residence Program. The program is organized to focus on facilitating the staff's creative process. The artists have been many. Some have stayed involved, others have contributed beautiful ideas and process and then gone on their way. One artist has created a fabric-painting kit, after gathering input from patients and nurses. The packages of T-shirts and paints captioned "Doodle Dabbler Paint Box Travelers," can be easily used while in bed and stored conveniently under the bed. Together, artists and nurses are testing what works and how best to implement the program.

Our musician, who has committed to work for a year, collaborates with nurses who are interested in using music as a nursing intervention, works with patients and families directly, and develops listening tapes for relaxation and guided imagery. His emphasis is on creating tapes of the patients' stories, accompanied with music, for the patients or for families who may lose a loved one during the hospitalization. Another musician plays the guitar for patients and their families, facilitating a songfest in which the nurses and physicians can join in. These representative examples indicate what is under way with current artists.

Some of the artists' perceptions of their experiences are enlightening. The next section describes the contributions and reactions of artists who have been directly involved in the Artists in Residence Program and of some individuals who have used art as a therapeutic process for themselves.

ARTISTS' PERCEPTIONS

As a patient and an artist, Darlene, a young woman, tapped her creative resources and empowered herself to become deeply involved in her own recovery from chronic pain. Diagnosed with fibromyalgia—a chronic, painful disease that had severely disabled her to the point that she became wheelchair-bound and severely depressed—she began a series of 72 drawings that she referred to as "the journey." The first was called *Pain.* After she became engaged in the drawing process, the colors, patterns, and symbols became important. Her drawings began to tell her story and guide her in new directions. The purple and orange represented her pain as she felt it, heart flowers in the landscapes were symbols of self-love, and the pathway drawn was the pathway of her journey. Darlene shared herself in her work.

> *My realization was that if I really wanted to help myself with the pain I knew I would have to change my whole life. It was in my drawings that I began to search for the person I was born to be.*

Her drawings reflected her experiences, her caretakers, and her relationship with her pain. The shared visual world was a potent and direct form of communication. She shared her drawings with her nurses and others as a vital part of her therapy and healing process. Darlene has now become involved with visiting patients in the hospital and sharing her experience of using art to help her own recovery process.

Leeann, who spent six months on the Bone Marrow Transplant Unit, shared her perceptions as an artist. Her experience arose directly from relationships with patients, families, and nursing staff. For months, this artist would visit individual patients in their hospital beds, exploring their interests and facilitating their involvement in a variety of art activities. She described one patient, "Michelle":

For months on end her world was a small, gray, antiseptic cubicle of filtered air, subdued light, fevers, chills, hair loss, vomiting, and pain—brief solitudes of despair and hope interrupted by the bustle of nurses, sometimes masked, gowned, and gloved. Their tirelessness was a match for her fatigue.

This sensitive and unique narrative conveyed her observations as she visited Michelle. After she left the hospital, Michelle sent the artist her own painting. Her "brushes" had been the toothettes (small, disposable cleaning instruments; cleaning her mouth, a seemingly trivial task, had been one of the most painful regimes of Michelle's care).

Subsequently, Leeann made Michelle's painting the central image of four portraits of Michelle as she had seen her during her hospital stay. Leeann was inspired by the relationship. She named this collective work, *Michelle's Flowers,* a reference to Michelle's painting of a bouquet of vividly colored flowers and a metaphor for Michelle in the four portraits. Leeann was able to share her experience of her relationship with Michelle by painting four sensitive portraits depicting the moods and feelings of Michelle that she had seen during her frequent visits.

I could only share my own joy and belief in creative expression as a healing process. Michelle always greeted me with a beautiful smile and strong but gentle gaze, testaments to her own healing process and gifts that I will forever cherish.

Michelle, during her hospitalization, valued the artist's interaction and participated by watching Leeann draw or listening to her talk about art. Sometimes, Leeann would simply listen. This artist was able to see the beauty in each patient's life and could interface with the nurses and their care. She was a witness to the process of Michelle's struggle to regain health.

What is left after blood counts, temperature readings, medications, and IV lines is a flower in all her humanness.

In another example, two women photographers formed a unique collaboration of photography. While one of the women endured treatment of breast cancer, they created together a photographic and written document of the treatment. The art dealt with and confronted creatively the experience of the woman living with the disease. Wanda, the patient, commented:

I want to be able to remember what has happened to me the last few months. Unlike some women I have read about who don't want to remember, I can never forget. The photographs and my journal will always be a link of me. The words provide an immediate and urgent release for what I'm feeling and the images document what I'm experiencing.

By exploring the uncharted territory of having breast cancer and documenting her healing journey, she felt she was coming out of the closet of social taboo and fear. She shared her humanity and her personal experience boldly. With her friend, who photographed her throughout her treatment, she created a powerful visual narrative.

CONCLUSION

Gabik (1991) encourages artists to evolve to new sets of ground rules for the future. Recovery is the willingness to make this system shift and create meaningful art. As Kaprow puts it: "Like art in which nothing is separate is a training in letting go of the separate self. . . . It is even possible that some lifelike art could become a discipline of healing . . . " (quoted in Galik, 1991). This is already happening. Nurses, doctors, patients, families, other health care providers, and artists are making a shift toward making art meaningful. It holds out hope for healing in the very environments that require it.

Mary Ann Winkler (1993) cheerfully reminded me, "One of my fondest memories as a child was when I was sick; my father brought me crayons. It used to always make me happy . . . . SO THINK CRAYONS!" How does one begin? Remember your childhood, and seek a memory of the freedom of your own creativity, long before you "learned" you were not good enough to be an "artist." That is your place to begin. Move from there to here-and-now, and paint your painting, write or tell your story, compose your poem, dance, play, laugh, and joyfully begin to sing your own song. I hope to persuade, inspire, and encourage other nurses to provide leadership and vision in this endeavor. As a nurse and as an artist, I see clearly that there is promise in the light.

REFERENCES

Arieh, S. (1976). *Creativity: The magic synthesis.* New York: Basic Books.

Bray, J. D. (1989). The relationships of creativity, time experience and mystical experience. New York University: CINAHL Abstract.

Burgess, A. W., & Hartman, C. R. (1993). Children's drawings. *Child-Abuse-Neglect, 17*(1), 161-168.

Capacchione, L. (1988). *The power of your other hand.* North Hollywood, CA: Newcastle Publishers.

Carper, B. A. (1978). Fundamental patterns of knowing in nursing. *Advances in Nursing Science, 1*(1), 13-23.

Chinn, P. L. (1985). Debunking myths in nursing theory and research. *Image: The Journal of Scholarly Inquiry, 17*(2), 45-49.

Chinn, P. L. (1989). Nursing patterns of knowing and feminist thought. *Nursing & Health Care, 10*(2), 71-75.

Chinn, P. L. (1991). *A phenomenologic/hermeneutic study of the art of nursing: Experiential interpretive criticism as method.* Proposal-in-progress, February 2.

Chinn, P. L., & Kramer, M. (1991). *Theory and nursing: A systematic approach* (3rd ed.). St. Louis: C. V. Mosby.

Coles, R. (1990). *The spiritual life of children.* Boston: Houghton Mifflin Co.

Csikszentmihalyi, M. (1990). *Flow.* New York: Harper & Row.

Edwards, B. (1986). *Drawing on the artist within.* New York: Simon & Schuster.

Gadamer, H. G. (1975). *Truth and method.* New York: Seabury.

Gabik, S. (1991). *The re-enchantment of art.* New York: Thames and Hudson.

Gaze, H. (1991). Lessons in creativity: Arts course for carers. *Nursing Times, 87*(34), 54-55.

Graham-Pole, J., Lane, M. T. R., & Rodrigue, R. (1992). *Art in the Bone Marrow Transplant Unit.* Proposal for Children's Miracle Network Grant.

Heidegger, M. (1977). *Basic writings.* New York: Harper & Row.

Highley, B., & Ferentz, T. (1988). *Esoteric inquiry.* New York: National League for Nursing.

Newman, M. (1986). *Health as expanding consciousness.* St. Louis: C. V. Mosby.

Nightingale, F. (1969). *Notes on Nursing: What it is, and what it is not.* New York: Dover Publications.

Polkinghorne, D. (1983). *Methodology for the human science: Systems of inquiry.* Albany, New York: State University of New York Press.

Updike, P. (1990). Music therapy results for ICU patients. *Dimensions of Critical Care Nurs., 9,* 39-45.

Updike, P. (1990). Through the lens of the artist-scientist: Reflections for the pediatric oncology nurse. *J. Pediatric Oncology Nursing, 7*(1), 4-8.

Van Manen, M. (1990). *Researching the lived experience.* Washington DC: Human Science for an Action Sensitive Pedagogy.

Watson, J. (1988). *Nursing: Human science and human care: A theory for nursing.* New York: National League for Nursing.

Watson, J. (1990). Caring knowledge and informed moral passion. *Advances in Nursing, 13*(1), 15-24.

Zukav, G. (1989). *The seat of the soul.* New York: Simon & Schuster.

BIBLIOGRAPHY

Camus, A. (1985). *The myth of sisyphus and other essays.* New York: Vintage Books.

Camus, A. (1986). *The plague.* New York: Random House, The Modern Library.

Dillard, A. (1982). *Pilgrim at tinker creek.* New York: Bantam Books.

Edwards, B. (1986). *Drawing on the artist within.* New York: Simon & Schuster.

Gadow, S. (1980). Body and self: A dialectic. *Journal of Medicine and Philosophy, 5,* 172–185.

Gadow, S. (1980). Existential advocacy: Philosophical foundation of nursing. In S. Spicker & S. Gadow (Eds.), *Nursing: Images and Ideals, opening dialogue with the humanities.* New York: Springer-Verlag.

Gadow, S. (1984). Touch and technology: Two paradigms of patient care. *Journal of Religion and Health, 23* (1).

Gadow, S. (1988). Covenant without cure: Letting go and holding on in chronic illness. In J. Watson & M. Ray (Eds.), *The Ethics of care and the ethics of cure: Synthesis and chronicity.* New York: National League for Nursing.

Gadow, S. (1993, April). *Women's health care: Social, medical, and ethical narratives.* Paper presented to the Conference on Women, Health Care, and Ethics. University of Tennessee, Knoxville, TN.

Gardner, H. (1982). *Art, mind and brain. A cognitive approach to creativity.* New York: Basic Books.

Ghiselin, B. (1953). *The creative process—A symposium.* Berkeley & Los Angeles, CA: University of California Press.

Merleau-Ponty, M. (1962). *Phenomenology of perception.* London: Routledge & Kegan Paul. [Translated from the French by Colin Smith].

Sartre, J. P. *Being and nothingness.* New York: Pocket Books, Washington Square Press.

11

Weaving Aesthetics into Practice: The Use of Aesthetic Techniques in Group Psychotherapy with Clients Remembering Repressed Traumatic Memories

Sharon Ann Cumbie
Sarah R. Rutherfoord

INTRODUCTION

Child Abuse

Child abuse has become a problem of great national, local, and individual concern. Abuse has far-reaching effects and is devastating to the developing child. It exerts a powerful, prolonged, and disruptive outcome on the individual. The psychosocial problems related to child abuse are long-term, touching on every stage of psychosocial development and self-concept. The client often presents to the health care system a complex set of complaints: low self-esteem, feelings of powerlessness, inability to trust, feelings of detachment, ineffective coping patterns, substance abuse, self-destructive patterns, and difficulty maintaining interpersonal relationships.

Common psychological mechanisms employed by children in their attempts to cope with the trauma include denial, emotional numbing, sublimation, dissociation, and repression. The predominant use of these coping styles, although successful in protecting the child during the abusive years, gives rise to an adult who has little insight into the relationship between childhood trauma and current life problems.

Repression and Remembering

Repression is a psychological defense mechanism whereby an individual blocks from the conscious mind events that are too painful and overwhelming for the person to consciously handle at the time of the event. The purpose of repression is pure and simple: protection. The memories may remain buried in the subconscious for a period of days, weeks, or years. Repression, then, is a form of amnesia in which the individual selectively blocks unmanageable memories. The result of this "selective amnesia" is a recollection of the past that is perceptually distorted.

De-repression is the process of connecting with the reality of the past and remembering the events of the past that have been repressed. The recollected memories are seldom clear or precise; more often, they are recalled as vague, hazy, dream-like pieces. Frequently, the survivor will be riddled with doubt regarding the validity of the memory.

The Healing Journey

The decision to heal is one of the most difficult steps taken in the process of recovering from childhood abuse. The early stages of healing are often filled with crises as the client begins to get in touch with the feelings associated with past trauma. If there is repression, the work of remembering these repressed traumatic memories and getting in touch with feelings associated with the past can become the most intense, painful, and consuming phase of the recovery process.

It is a fragile period in the healing journey, and the task of the therapist is to structure the recovery experience in such a way as to balance the exploration of painful memories and feelings with a stabilizing and integrative period. A pattern of remembering and then coping with the memory, as opposed to dwelling continuously on the emerging memory, seems to allow the client to remain relatively well-integrated while doing this delicate and painful work.

Aesthetic as Process

The aesthetic is a pattern of knowing that focuses on meaning and the expression of meaning. The aesthetic is a creative way of knowing in which the knower can envision possibilities that transcend time and space, thus exploring and discovering new knowledge (Carper, 1978; Chinn, 1987). This way of knowing allows the knower to appreciate alternative perceptions, to comprehend the depth of these perceptions, and to ultimately communicate this new knowledge through creative expression.

An important element of the aesthetic process is creativity. Creativity is not the same as art. Not everyone is capable of becoming a great artist, but all persons are creative, no matter how limited (Barron, 1968). Barron stated that "because we are capable of reflecting upon ourselves, we are committed to an artistic enterprise in the creation of our own personality" (p. 56). Wadeson (1980) proposed that the creative experience allows one to escape oneself and suggests a kind of transcendent process, a feeling of touching and being part of a more universal experience than the unique conditions of one's own life. She further suggested that, through the creative process, a profound understanding of oneself is obtained and that "integration" is probably the result of the interface of the personal and the universal.

During the healing process, the client becomes consciously aware of the repressed, unconscious events of childhood trauma. Aesthetic techniques in psychotherapy utilize the creative process in facilitating the work of remembering and coping with painful and disturbing memories. The aesthetic process offers the client a more gentle, metaphorical pathway to a knowledge of the self by providing an avenue of expression for the intense, emotionally charged memories that surface, as well as a record of the process. Aesthetics provides a medium for letting the subconscious speak and facilitates an individual's expression of feelings, but does not seem to elicit the same negative responses of fear and anxiety as does the more traditional approach of direct confrontation with the self.

The utilization of drawing and writing in a journaling process allows the client to access and record the emerging pieces of memory with the confidence that, because the information is permanently recorded, the process can be "put aside" without the risk of forgetting this newly remembered information. These pieces of memory can be methodically gathered within the context and process of journaling and pieced together at the client's own pace.

THE METHOD

In this section, techniques for incorporating aesthetics into the therapeutic process are presented, along with reflections on the experience of this creative process. The techniques described are in the context of group psychotherapy that utilizes aesthetic techniques within the group psychodynamic process.

The Group Structure

Psychotherapy with a group of individuals who have experienced childhood abuse requires a considerable amount of structure during the developing stages of the group, because of the trust issues and the control needs of this particular client population. Adherence to a routine structure for the group sessions, giving predictability to the group process, allows participants a feeling of safety. Two-hour sessions seem to provide adequate time for sharing journal work and engaging in group process. The ideal number for this type of group is eight persons. There are three twelve-week sessions each year, beginning in the fall and continuing through winter and spring. Breaks are taken during the Christmas and Easter seasons and the entire summer quarter. The summer break allows participants to experiment with new skills and "take a breather" from their hard work. It also provides the therapist some respite time.

Each group session begins with a basic check-in: participants share briefly how their week has been and present issues or themes for later discussion. During the first group of each quarter, group rules are developed and explicated by both therapist and members. All following group sessions proceed in the same manner: check-in (20–30 minutes), sharing of homework assignments (30 minutes), a short break (10 minutes), group process time (40 minutes), and wrap-up (10 minutes). The adherence to a schedule encourages participants to address issues in a more open and relevant manner and discourages their holding back sharing feelings or engaging in the group process. Starting each group session with check-in usually sets the tone of the group process phase of the session. Sharing participant experiences with the homework assignments in the Creative Process Journal provides reinforcement for those who did the assignment and allows members to learn about the ways in which others engage in an aesthetic process.

The experience of coming together in a group provides an opportunity for members to develop several areas of life skills. As group cohesion develops, members are able to explore issues of trust as they enter into relationship with one another. The sharing of common experiences of childhood helps each member to realize that he or she is not alone and isolated in these experiences, thus reducing personal shame and self-blaming. The group experience also offers a venue for trying out and practicing new behaviors, such as genuine expression of feelings and appropriate confrontation. The group ultimately offers a safe environment where, often for the first time, the individual's experience is validated and accepted.

As I started to feel safe in my support group, facilitated by
a licensed therapist specializing in abuse recovery work, I

*could share verbally the details of my own childhood trau-
mas. I was believed! No one tried to change the subject because it was distressing to hear my abuse history. The group
members were able to mirror back to me, through their facial and verbal expressions and emotional reactions, what I
had up until this time not allowed my subconscious to feel
or express.*

*The turning point in my recovery was set in motion by the
permission the group gave me to tell them my memories no
matter how gruesome or disgusting they were. This is an in-
valuable gift, encouraging an incredible drive to heal and a
comforting knowledge that I was definitely not crazy. They
knew I did not make it up. I had been bumping up against
life in a normal manner for someone who had lived my
circumstances.*

*So many of our reactions to our individualized traumas
were the same. When we would come to group to present
our common assignments, it never ceased to amaze me how
similar were our depictions of a given subject matter. None
of us collaborated on the execution of our work. This phenomenon validated for me the accuracy of my memories.*

The Creative Process Journal

The Creative Process Journal is a notebook in which the client
records thoughts, feelings, remembrances, hopes, ideas, or anything that is a part of the healing journey. Recordings may be verbal, poetic, or visual representation. All homework assignments
are done in this book. The journal, then, becomes an extremely
personal accounting of each person's individual progress. The
journal is often described by clients as feeling like an extension of
themselves. This feeling of "bonding" helps to enhance the meaning of the journaling process as a coping strategy.

Clients are provided structured exercises, utilizing techniques
such as drawing, collage, poetry, and metaphorical storytelling,
during the initial stages of the therapeutic process. This helps
to facilitate their becoming comfortable with aesthetic methods
of recording information and processing their feelings. These

aesthetic techniques enable the client to work metaphorically, with images, rather than attempt a literal representation of a feeling or emotion, which is often impossible to do. Once a significant degree of comfort with these techniques is achieved, less structure is necessary; clients increasingly demonstrate using the process in their own unique way.

The journal offers a permanent representation of their journey. The advantage of this permanence is that the contents of reflection, once recorded in the journal, are not subject to the distortions of memory. These recorded pieces of information are particularly helpful in identifying patterns and providing the puzzle pieces of emerging memories. Additionally, the journal becomes a tangible object. It is often easier for a client to discuss difficult feelings or remembrances by relating to a picture or a poem created in the journal.

> *The practice of "journaling" gave me unexpected peace of mind. The journal is an extension of me, a safe place to permanently store the horrors, confusion, and memories—it is my confidant and friend who allows me to explore my memories and feelings in a haphazard fashion without even a shred of criticism or judgment.*
>
> *To my astonishment, journaling tapped into a creative part of me, long ago abandoned, releasing a stream of healing energy that ebbed and flowed but moved forever forward. I could not have turned back. I could have stopped dead in the water with my bow snugly cradled in the forward movement of my healing currents, but resolutely unable to turn away from my innate mission.*
>
> *Another benefit I derived from journaling was the unquestioned clarity of the facts and events in my life that shaped who I am and what I felt, saw, heard, learned, reacted to, and survived. I could let go of the distorted justifications and lies my parents forced on me to vindicate their deviant behavior.*
>
> *My journals have been so important to my recovery that if my house were to catch on fire, after getting my children out, I would race to extricate them to safety.*

Materials

Through experimentation and sometimes strong feedback from group members, the following materials are suggested for beginning this work:

- A spiral-bound (side-, *not* top-bound! this seems to make a big difference) standard size (8½" × 11") drawing notebook. Acid-free paper is encouraged; the extra cost is minimal for far greater permanence.
- Box of 24 color crayons.
- Box of 8 jumbo marking pens, standard colors.
- Bottle of school glue (e.g., Elmer's all-purpose glue).
- Glue stick.
- Paper scissors.
- Large manila envelope to store magazine and newspaper cut-out images for collage.

Starting with simple art supplies helps to reduce anxiety about working with "art materials" and also seems to ease tapping into the "child within." As comfort levels increase, other materials may be added, such as oil pastels, tempera paints, or watercolors, but generally the initial supplies remain sufficient. The addition of a set of fine-tipped pens/markers is helpful for achieving greater detail in drawings.

STRUCTURING THE WORK

Becoming Comfortable with the Process

Initially, the therapist may encounter resistance to these aesthetic methods from clients who are anxious about engaging in an activity that seems like "art." It is important to emphasize that this is not art, in the formal sense, but only another method of self-expression. The greatest barrier to clients' engaging in an aesthetic process is the general mystique that surrounds artistic endeavor and the belief that only a chosen few are capable of doing creative work. Emphasis on the process instead of the product seems to allow clients to overcome feelings of self-consciousness and resistance.

Clients are instructed in the following techniques for beginning their work:

1. Find a quiet place where you will not be disturbed.
2. Lay out your art supplies in front of you so that they are readily available.
3. Close your eyes for a moment, take in a few deep, cleansing breaths, and tell yourself, "Relax, relax."
4. Read your assignment and reflect quietly for a moment on what it means to *you*. Remember, there is no right or wrong way to do the assignment.
5. Let go of the "thinking" part of your mind and just allow the process to take hold. Don't try to analyze what you are doing, just allow the spontaneity of the moment to take over.
6. After you finish your piece, give it a title and date it. Reflect on the meaning the piece has for you, and write a statement about its meaning.
7. Do not allow yourself to engage in criticizing the quality of the work you have done. Focus on the completion of the *process,* not on the outcome of the *product.*

Initially, providing nonthreatening assignments, such as Capaccione's (1979) "What's in a Name" or "Parts of Self" exercises, facilitates the client in becoming both familiar and comfortable with the process. Assignments can then be structured to reflect the current issues and themes of the group process. (A list of texts useful for creating these assignments is provided at the end of this chapter.)

Working through the Stages of Healing

There are stages in the healing journey. Like other psychodynamic processes, these stages are seldom experienced in a linear manner;

more often, they occur in a convolutional pattern. The metaphor of psychodynamic process being like "peeling the layers of an onion" is appropriate for the patterns found in healing from child abuse.

Identification of the following major stages can be useful in structuring the aesthetic work for the group: Making the decision to heal; identifying the impact of the abuse; getting in touch with feelings; learning how to feel; dealing with the anger; letting go of shame and blame; nurturing the child within; remembering the past; taking care of self; integrating; and healing. Examples of how aesthetic technique can be utilized to facilitate work during these stages will be presented in the remainder of the chapter.

Awareness of the Long-Term Effects of Abuse

An important stage in the healing journey is the process in which the client gains awareness of how past childhood experiences have affected and continue to affect his or her life as an adult. Clients are provided general information regarding the purported long-term effects of childhood abuse and are facilitated to share, during group discussion, specific examples from their lives. Journal exercises to help explicate these relationships are provided in an attempt to further develop clients' awareness. This new knowledge seems to have an empowering effect on individuals as they begin to see problem areas in their lives as having been externally influenced and not as part of their genuine core being (Figures 1–3).

> *The long-term effects of incest on the adult are profound. The betrayal and the other emotional sequelae would affect and impact my life so massively I would become crippled in my ability to sustain a healthy intimate relationship on a sexual or emotional level with my husband and on an emotional level with more than one female friend at a time. Luckily, I was able to create and maintain an emotionally intimate, nurturing, stable relationship with my children— a skill I worked very hard to accomplish and from which I have derived much joy and a feeling of success.*

Figure 1. "Abuse Incarnate"
The agony of the abuse was stored in my gut, hidden. It had been transformed into a more socially acceptable response to the injury and grief of my childhood experience.

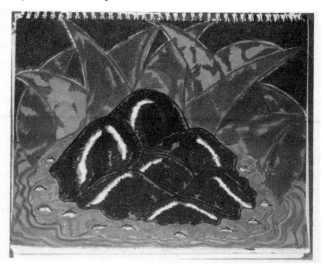

Figure 2. "The Ninja: Embodied Pain Healing From the Inside Out"
Once I had drawn this mental image of the emotions I was feeling, these images became meaningful messages of the internal environment of my body.

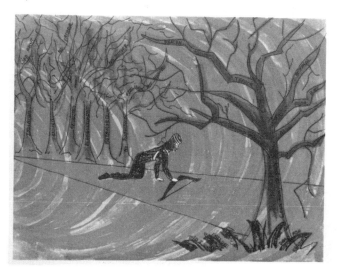

Figure 3. "Photos of Colon: Clinical Evidence of the Body's Wisdom" The two drawings of my intestines shown here were done almost a year before having the colonoscopy. I was amazed to see evidence of the embodied knowledge I had accessed. It was affirming of the value of the creative process.

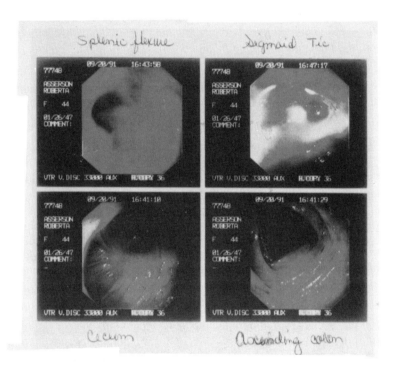

These drawings represent a sample of journal work that allowed me to see the magnitude of the effects of child abuse on the well being of my body. I knew, without a doubt that the pain I had internalized had caused my disease. Once in touch with this realization, I began to get better. I began to heal.

Phobias developed due to the frequent and intense abuses suffered for too many years. These fears are each directly connected with specific traumas. The phobias that I have carried into my adult life and which have the most tenacity had originated as a coping strategy for survival while I was younger and still unable to leave my parents' home.

With the support of the therapists and group members, I have attempted to be more patient with these sequelae and myself. Feeling freer to express my anger at my parents for creating an environment where these handicaps could take root, and really looking at and sharing these unfortunate experiences with people who believed me, has loosened the grasp these phobias have had.

Life Line: *My initial reaction upon being given this assignment was, "How is this going to help me feel better? This is just busy work." This assignment had an unexpected impact on me. It was the first time I realized there were large memory blackouts in my life; that I was not skilled in knowing what my feelings were and that I had a great deal of what was for me at the time very scary memory work to do.*

Feelings Work

After decades of emotional numbing, getting in touch with one's feeling can be like anesthesia giving way to throbbing pain after dental surgery. This stage of healing requires much time and frequent revisiting. The client must learn not only to identify *what* he or she is feeling, but also to deal appropriately with often intense and emotionally charged new states of being. This is one of the phases in which the metaphorical qualities of the aesthetic process are greatly appreciated by the client. The process offers a tool for coping with sometimes overwhelming feelings.

Being able to give a guise to my feelings provided me with a reassuring way to keep in touch with and identify them. I view them as old comfortable friends now instead of strange or frightening entities. Having these emotions

*represented in my journal is like having a photo album full
of relatives. Some are fun and easy to be around and some
are disruptive, but they all belong to me whether I take
pleasure in them or not. It is healthier for me to be aware of
them than to have continued an anesthetized or ghostlike
existence. I find I have far more rational control over my
rage and anger, not inflicting [them] inappropriately on
others, subsequent to drawing them (these emotions) in my
journal.*

*One of the first assignments I was given by the group
therapist was to go over a* Feelings Chart. *Once again I
thought rather smugly, "Of course I can feel; I cry and laugh,
don't I, at appropriate times." Little did I know how numb I
really was. Forced to realistically define how I felt at a given
time whether it be while working on the life-line (past feelings) or how I was feeling today, I began to get in touch with
how I really felt. The most important insight I learned was
how shut down I was and that it was all right to feel. In fact,
to feel promoted healing and a sense of true mental health
for the first time in my life.*

*The Feelings Chart became as essential a tool to moving
ahead in my recovery as learning the multiplication tables
in the fourth grade is to going on to higher math and understanding it. If I didn't learn those monstrous times tables, I
simply couldn't learn any more math; I could not even fake
it. If I didn't learn how to feel and identify what I was feeling, I couldn't move forward. I would be dead in the water.*

*While doing my feelings-work, I began to connect feelings
with certain colors I used in my Art Journal. After four
months of intense feelings identification work, I had one of
my first flashback dreams. Another surprise for me. I found
myself wanting to flee, to turn back, to be numb again. I
coped with the help of my new tools, "journaling," my facilitated support group, and my books on healing from abuse.*

Remembering: Self-Knowledge, Piece by Piece

The work of getting in touch with the effects of the past and of
identifying and coping with feelings prepares the client for the

next stage in the recovery process: remembering repressed traumatic memories. It is important to be mindful of the fact that this remembering process is not something the client "decides to do," but is part of the healing process, occurring naturally *when the client is emotionally ready.*

These memories are most often remembered in bits and pieces, which can be very frustrating. This fragmented way of remembering allows one to gradually incorporate the memories of these past traumas into conscious awareness, thus protecting the individual from being overwhelmed, and potentially retraumatized, by the remembered events.

The aesthetic process can be most useful during this stage in providing the client with techniques that facilitate recording and processing these memories. Often, although the intensity of feelings associated with the memory is beyond words, the individual is able to capture the essence of the experience through the images of the drawings. Clients report that working in their journals during these remembering episodes can be "grounding": it keeps them in touch with tangible reality. The recorded image also provides a permanent piece of the "puzzle of self" (Figures 4-6).

I could acknowledge my past with what seemed to me unquestionable clarity when first embarking on this journey in July, 1989. Unknown to my cognitive brain was the fact that there were buried memories, with a power all their own, driving me to face the reality of where I had come from and where I needed to go.

Parts of Me: *In order to clear my mind enough to start acknowledging my past, I had to honestly identify who I truly was at that precise moment. Doing the Parts Of Me exercises facilitated this clarification very well.*

Deciding to face the memories was about as inviting as jumping into the green slime-lined swimming pool at Camp Kiwanianna on a freezing cold summer morning and being forced to swim laps. I soon decided I was as ready as anyone can be who has to do something scary. After all, it's only a "memory" of a real trauma. I had already physically survived; now all that was left was to remember and deal with whatever repressed feelings accompany the memories.

Figure 4. "Overwhelmed"
Naked in the spirals, caught between the innate need to break the silence and the fear of loosing both my immediate and extended family. I knew I must break the bonds of silence, whatever the cost, in order to heal. Is the pain of the loss going to be less than the pain of the silence?

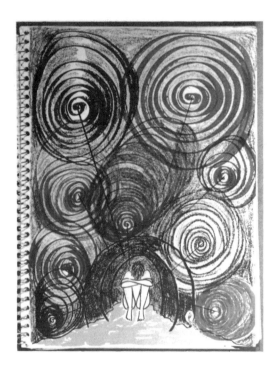

Unknown to my cognitive brain was the fact that there was buried memories with a power all their own driving me to face the reality of where I had come from and where I needed to go. Connections were made with the pain that I had dissociated through much of my childhood. I had been in possession of only dim fragments of my life, until now.

Figure 5. "Cast Out into a Motherless Vaccume"
I felt imprisoned between dusk and dawn, constantly trying to open a door without hinges. I felt alienated from the world as a child. Fortunately, I had been given a glimpse of a softer, more nurturing world by a loving aunt and uncle. Their love was like a beacon of light, giving me hope and enabling me to survive.

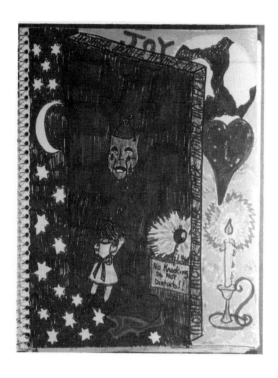

Figure 6. "My Father's Blessing"
This was the first time I allowed myself to encounter the horror and suffocating pain of my childhood. It came crashing back in full force, causing a purging and cleansing of my soul, extricating me with its healing power from the abyss. I was able to break down walls that allowed me to go on with my healing process.

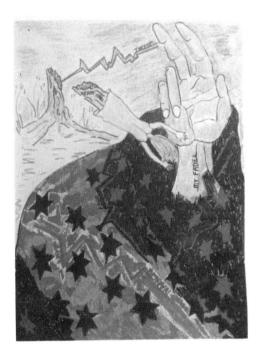

After three months had passed and I was becoming comfortable with the emerging process, group, and observing that indeed you wouldn't melt away like the wicked witch in Dorothy's Oz from a flashback, I started to have pictorial fragments of memories slam into my consciousness while I slept, always preceded by my own voice alerting me in an urgent manner to listen, watch, and remember what it was going to show me.

Some of the fragments were riddles to me but I knew they were veracious (truthful) and essential to my healing and so recorded them in my journal. Their appearance created ambivalence in me. On the one hand, they were terrifying (as any unknown phenomenon is), but on the other, they were substantiating my progress.

The time span for all of the cognate fragments to be pieced together correctly ranged from a few weeks to fourteen months. Some are still not clear, but I do not dwell on them; they will come together in time, when I am able to handle the memory and not before.

If I hadn't recorded these scraps of images (including all the colors they wore) and dated them, I feel like I might have lost their significance in a sea of disarray, slowing down my healing process. By journaling I could divert all the energy used to try and hold on to what I remembered (without its support) to a more depleted part or parts of me. Having the many puzzle pieces all laid out in front of me made it possible for me to realize the abuses that actually took place.

Integration: Pulling It All Together

The group often echoes a phrase: "Getting well feels like going crazy." Each stage in the healing journey brings an increased awareness of the past and the relationship of the past to the present. Traumatic memories are remembered and incorporated into the whole being. A gradual process of empowerment occurs. The individual becomes confident in his or her ability to manage and cope with the memories of the past, the events of the present, and the potential for the future.

Integration signals the completion of a cycle within the process of healing. The group will often take respite in the themes of integration and healing before delving into a deeper layer of the healing journey, in which a new cycle begins. Integration is a period of reflection, of putting the pieces together, and of acknowledging the hard work that has been completed. It is a time of affirmation, with a resulting confidence in the process that is being mastered (Figures 7 and 8).

Figure 7. "Piggy's Field: The First Meeting"
Meeting my inner child for the first time was frightening. She was so needy, neglected, isolated and waiting. I looked her in the eye, recognizing her little face as mine. I gave her the stuffed animal, Piggy, and assured her that I would be back when I was stronger and able to open myself to know and cherish her.

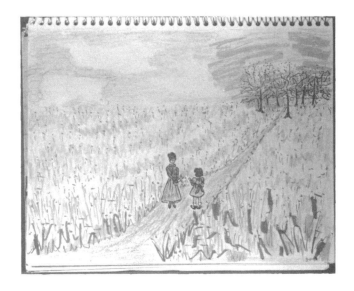

A turning point for me was when I was finally able to embrace the child within me. I had avoided this for a long time because I was afraid of her pain. But then I realized it was up to me to parent her.

We work well together. I support her healing and help her when she is afraid or lonely. She has helped me to learn to play, to lighten up a bit. We heal a little more each day.

Figure 8. "I am Free, A Victim No More!"
The key to success is self-care and picking a safe, non-threatening environment. I no longer set myself up for failure. For all my life, I blamed myself for what I had experienced as a child. Now I am free of the blame and the shame. I am free to just BE.

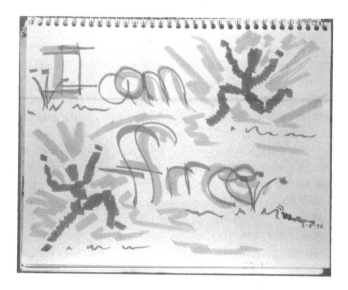

Rejoice in your newly found voice; I did. Luckily for my family I had a support group to go to and had made some telephone friends of fellow survivors so we would exercise our newly found loquaciousness with each other, relieving our families of having to hear about our abuse work and experiences.

My teen-age daughter described how she felt when she would hear even a small amount of details. "Yuk, it is like picking someone else's nose to listen to all of that unhappy talk."

What I am saying is be selective. (It's a skill survivors need to practice.) Our families hurt for us so they need a little time out and room that's free from listening to abuse stories; respect their boundaries.

I have found that by not always using avoidance to cope with unwanted fears they begin to lose some of their strength each time I am successful in overcoming the anxiety. The key to these successes is self-care and picking a safe, nonthreatening environment. I no longer set myself up for failure.

CONCLUSION

This brief overview has presented the utilization of aesthetic process within group psychotherapy with survivors of childhood abuse. Select examples of how aesthetics was incorporated into this process were given, to provide the reader with a general idea of how aesthetic process can be woven into one's practice. The aesthetic way of knowing offers a gentle pathway for coming to know the self and for integrating painful feelings or memories into one's conscious awareness. In addition, a healing effect seems to be achieved from the process of engaging in creative activity that is separate from the psychodynamic process.

Variations of this method have been used with children, adolescents, and adults, with multiple treatment and intervention aims, and with mental health, medical, and spiritual concerns and processes. Aesthetic methods are readily available to nurses and are appropriate in supporting such nursing goals as promoting holistic healing and facilitating human well-being.

. . . When I reflect on the method of healing I have experienced, a metaphorical vision of the process comes to mind. It is not unlike the sciences of paleontology and archaeology. Instead of geological layers, I had to carefully and meticulously uncover the layers of buried feelings, needs, and memories. Piecing the shards of my broken authentic self together was like the archeologist who reassembles broken pieces of the broken pottery, all the while recording these small artifacts in a record book, drawing, photographing and describing them through writing, in an attempt to describe this lost civilization. The tools used in this archeological process are also metaphorically the same ones utilized through this aesthetic method of recovery. Sometimes I

needed a spade and pick ax, other times I used a soft brush and gloves, gently winnowing out the negative messages and patterns of behavior of my life through my sifting screen, carrying the healthy skills away in my bucket. All of this was done so I could recover my lost history and reconstruct the sequence of my life. I became free to emotionally bond with my fellow human beings, myself, and more deeply to my God.

REFERENCES

Barron, F. (1968). *Creativity and personal freedom*. New York: John Wiley & Sons.

Capaccione, L. (1979). *The Creative Journal*. Athens, OH: Swallow Press/Ohio University Press.

Carper, B. (1978). Fundamental patterns of knowing in nursing. *Advances in Nursing Science, 1,* 13-24.

Chinn, P. (1987). Nursing's patterns of knowing and feminist thought. *Nursing and Health Care, 10*(2), 71-75.

Wadeson, H. (1980). *Art psychotherapy*. New York: John Wiley & Sons.

RECOMMENDED TEXTS

Adamson, E. (1990). *Art as healing*. Boston: Conventure.

Furth, G. M. (1988). *The secret world of drawings: Healing through art*. Boston: Sigo Press.

Kandinsky, W. (1977). *Concerning the spiritual in art*. New York: Dover.

Kent, C., & Stewars, J. (1992). *Learning by heart: Teachings to free the creative spirit*. New York: Bantam Books.

London, P. (1989). *No more secondhand art: Awakening the artist within*. Boston: Shambhala Press.

Richards, M. C. (1989). *Centering in pottery, poetry, and person*. Middletown, CT: Wesleyan University Press.

12

The Seeing Self: Photography and Storytelling as a Health Promotion Methodology

Mary Koithan

I feel out of touch with the rhythms and meanings of my own existence. I feel a need to sit quietly with myself and my world. . . . I need to get in touch with my life forces, my energy source, whatever gives me my being. . . . I feel a need to "see" myself and learn to quiet myself so that I can comprehend, understand, and hear [my world]. (Koithan, 1988)

*I*n the current technocratic world, the human experience of life is seldom, if ever, questioned. People become consumed with the need for more advanced, more complex, and faster communication and transportation. Human life quickly becomes a harried flow of existence, often devoid of meaning and purpose. Interpersonal relationships are technologically rather than humanly dependent, and people begin to assume the faceless nature of the computerized, mechanized world in which we live.

Yet, timeless insight into the nature of human beings points to every person's innate desire to seek meaning in life's experiences. All major world religions and spiritual groups speak to the necessity of understanding self, the God-in-me, the immortal (Bach, 1977, 1988; Kafka, 1972; Prabhavananda, 1948). Therefore, to pursue modern life as it is currently experienced is, in part, contrary to the essential nature of the human being and creates a schism between I/me. This schism, which can be described in terms of harmony/disharmony between the perceived/ideal self and the realized/experienced self, results in perceptions of disarray, anxiety, and disease (Watson, 1988, 1993). These perceptions are borne out in epidemiological statistics of stress disorders, indicating that today's world is directly responsible for an increased incidence of and mortality from diseases related to environmental and personal stress (Center for Disease Control, 1992).

To alter the perceived disharmony between the ideal self and the self as daily experienced or lived, methodologies are needed that assist persons in assigning meaning, interpreting events, and illuminating purpose. Techniques that enhance the "self as seeing" need to be incorporated daily as means by which people seek health and prevent disease. These particular activities serve to empower the human spirit while calming the "noise" of the battering world.

Aesthetic methodologies are uniquely able to facilitate healing between the ideal and perceived self. Aesthetic knowing defies translation of personal meaning into words (Carper, 1978). Genuine meaning, which is necessary for the exploration of the I/me schism, is believed to be lost when translated into verbal and written communication. Aesthetic modes of awareness deliver meaning to the soul, bringing images of healing and health into explicit awareness and unifying the self as perceived.

The aesthetic healing modality of photography, coupled with self-reflection and storytelling, is particularly useful in illuminating purpose and meaning in the human experience of life. In those moments of seeing self as purposeful, the inherent I/me wholeness is recaptured and healing occurs.

Photography serves to narrow the world as seen. There is a tendency in daily life to internalize the entire visual horizon. We take all of its noise, confusion, and mechanization into our being and elevate it to a level of significance wherein "it" becomes "us." The enormity of this life quickly overwhelms us, and we soon lose effectiveness in daily activities as well as our sense of purpose and direction. The camera's lens selects areas of concern on which to focus and concentrate. Thoughts and feelings are narrowed. We become less scattered and, through this, gain a sense of empowerment and calm, of personal well-being and health.

Sitting quietly with thoughts permits self-reflection and the construction of meaning through storytelling. As we listen, we are often aware of the disjointed multitude of thoughts that constantly bombard our minds. As vision is focused through the camera's lens and thoughts are directed toward the meaning of life through self-reflection, the disjointed becomes one; mind, body, and spirit become connected.

PERSONAL MEANING AS HEALTH

The idea of health in literature has been examined by many authors. Health broadly defined is "any state of optimal functioning, well-being, or progress." Well-being is defined as "happiness." The act of healing is the process of health promotion and restoration. Heal is further defined as "to become whole and sound" (American heritage dictionary, 1980). The etymological roots of the word are in the Anglo-Saxon word "haelen," which means to become whole (Keller, 1981; Quinn, 1989; Smith, 1990).

Smith (1983) reviewed literature relevant to the current conceptualizations of health and developed four models of health: (1) the clinical model: health as the absence of disease; (2) the role performance model: health as the ability to conform to social norms and expectations; (3) the adaptive model: health as determined by the person's ability to interact "fruitfully" and effectively within constantly changing natural and social environments; and (4) the eudaemonistic model: health as the ideals of general well-being and self-realization (Smith, 1983). Smith claimed that the models are not mutually exclusive; rather, they are alternative models of health, and each holds validity. Each model presents a distinctive frame of reference and distinctive goals, and thus would precipitate distinctive health promotion and healing modalities by individuals. Further, each model would promote different types of intervention and care from the health care system. Smith concluded that the models may actually formulate a "progressive expansion of the idea of health" wherein individuals are viewed "within broader and broader contexts" (Smith, 1983, p. 89).

Newman (1979) claimed that there is another view of health wherein "disease is a manifestation of health" (Newman, 1979, p. 9). A hallmark of the conceptualization of health and health promotion from this perspective is the belief that health and illness "should be equally viewed as expressions of the life processes" (Rogers, 1970, p. 10). Life processes described from these theoretical perspectives stress the interwoven web of relationships that humans have with the totality of the universe (Newman, 1979; Parse, 1987; Rogers, 1970; Watson, 1985). Health then becomes the process of unfolding within the human–environmental relationship (Parse, 1990b). It is a creative process of becoming, of harmonizing the explicate and implicate orders of reality within the individual as consciousness unfolds or expands (Grof, 1985; Newman, 1979; Parse, 1990a). Thus, the person is healed or whole, experiencing a sense of oneness, connection, or human well-being.

This model of health is unlike any described by Smith (1983). It relies on "space/time/energy and consciousness expansion . . . and [conceptualizes] health as awareness . . . and personal empowerment" (Meleis, 1991, p. 112). Health as a manifestation of the implicate order of field patterning is an emergent, lived experience of the individual and is assigned positions and definitions of value and worth based on the individual's understanding, life experiences, and language. Health as process and health promotion as facilitation of human empowerment and human awareness embrace the notion that human beings are inherently one with the ideal, the infinite order. Health promotion occurs as meanings unfold, human purpose is examined and illuminated, and alternatives take wing.

Health can be promoted as alternatives in explanation are explored, understanding of the implicate order of reality is expanded, and awareness of the possibilities and the nature of implicate order is enhanced. When human beings understand the nature of the explicate order as reflective of the whole, assign meaning and value to their own life's rhythmical patterning with its seeming paradoxes of harmony/disharmony, order/disorder, and pleasant/unpleasant, and transcend what is to what is not yet, they begin to realize and cherish the unitary nature of their realized and ideal selves, placing them in right relationship with the universal order and giving them ultimate purpose and value in life. This transcendent movement of the person embraces that which is but is not yet realized, and entails an expansion of human awareness which is both implicit and explicit. "Movement is seen as an awareness of self" toward a sense of one's own on boundarylessness and timelessness that is reflective of the pandimensional nature of the implicate order (Newman, 1979, p. 72). Health promotion and healing, from this transformative perspective, form a model of human empowerment rather than human control.

This model of health, health promotion, and healing is consistent with a changing scientific and paradigmatic perspective that has been heralded by a growing number in the scientific community (Bohm, 1980, 1985, 1987; Grof, 1985, 1988a, 1988b, 1990; Newman, Sime, & Corcoran-Perry, 1991; Rogers, 1970, 1990, 1993). The philosophical tenets concerning the nature of reality, epistemological systems, and the metaphysical are currently being challenged by dramatic discoveries in the disciplines of physics and mathematics and in the human sciences of psychology, anthropology, and nursing. Current research in many scientific disciplines has "shattered the very foundations of the Newtonian model of the universe" (Grof, 1985, p. 53). Absolute time and space, the solid nature of the universe, the definitions of laws and unchangeable principles of solid matter, the deterministic-objective system of phenomena and description—all were significantly challenged by the discipline of physics in the early 1900s. Consciousness research in psychology and psychiatry during the mid-1900s continued the challenge of linear time and space, causal events, and separatism that hallmarked mechanistic science. Individuals reported that past and future appeared to be intimately related to present events. Energy patterns replaced the solid nature of the universe, and boundaries were seen as less absolute and more fluid (Grof, 1985). Quantum physics suggested that the meaning of nature and reality can only be understood through careful study of the patterns of relationships and interconnections (Grof, 1985).

The emergent paradigm can be described as holistic and concerned with the unique human phenomenon as experienced by the individual. A closed attitude toward phenomenal interpretation is rejected by human science; an "engaged" and open approach to the analysis of phenomenal experience is instead the desired outcome (Giorgi, 1970). Paternalistic attitudes of categorization, reductionism, and manipulation are inconsistent with the new world-view (Watson, 1985b). All phenomena are viewed as "unified self-organizing fields embedded into a larger self-organizing field . . . which is identified by pattern" and unitary interaction with the larger whole (Newman et al., 1991). Change is characterized as unidirectional, unpredictable movement leading to greater complexity in organization—an "unfolding" (Newman et al., 1991, p. 4).

Each person is a holographic reflection of the implicate patterning of the whole, and manifestations holographically reflect this same pattern. Humans change their interpretations of the reflections as they understand more specifically the nature of the implicate order and the nature of their individual reflection of the implicate order, and begin to expand their cognitive and precognitive awareness of the meaning of the implicate order (Newman, 1986; Rogers, 1990a; Watson, 1985a). Health promotion, then, becomes an activity whereby the individual can change interpretations of the explicate order in order to see more clearly the perfect holographic reflection that is his or her life. As the realized self becomes more aware that it holistically reflects the implicate order and that its individual life is reflective of expanding, diversifying, universal fields of patterning, paths to understanding human purpose and universal placement open, human possibilities are transcended, harmony is perceived, understanding is expanded, and health is promoted (Parse, 1990b; Rogers, 1970, 1986, 1988, 1993; Watson, 1985a, 1985b).

Health promotion and healing activities within unitary–transformative science embrace the experiences of the person as lived and are celebrated as reflections of the mystical, unknowable, implicate order. They are not specific interventive strategies with a predetermined end product. "To intervene with a specific solution in mind is to say we know what form the pattern is taking" (Newman, 1986, p. 68). Because the person lives freely the possibilities and the underlying pattern is continually diversifying, that which is not yet remains a universal mystery (Parse, 1993; Watson, 1989). Therefore, health promotion and healing activities are defined by each person as those strategies that enhance individualized understanding and pattern recognition.

Pattern is recognized through multiple modes of awareness that include empirical, ethical, personal, and aesthetic patterns of recognition and knowing (Carper, 1978). Aesthetic knowledge is particularly important to the understanding of concepts and meanings that are not easily translated into verbal and written communication. Often, the meaning and definition of patterning are lost, because of inherent languaging discrepancies, in the words through which they are intended to be communicated. Intention, essence, and connotation held in personal meaning defy current empirical expression. In contrast, understanding is augmented through arts such as poetry, painting, sculpture, music, and photography. The difference primarily is one of perception rather than recognition. Perception unifies ends and means, leading to understanding and ultimately to action (Carper, 1978).

AESTHETICS AS A HEALTH PROMOTION MODALITY

Health promotion is the process by which persons examine and come to understand their unique life events as a reflection of the holonomic patterning, the universal, the ideal. As such, people cherish self, gain personal perspective and meaning, and evolve/ transcend their conscious being-in-this-world. Multiple modes of personal discovery enhance the person's ability to see self. Each person defines a personal way of contemplation and "seeing." As one discovers modality, aesthetics aid in the person's ability to translate perceptions that defy description and verbalization. Aesthetic modalities capture the essences of personal existence that resist empirical knowing.

Life cannot be "deductively known but inductively experienced" (Giorgi, 1970, p. 16). Human understanding must incorporate aesthetics, beauty, and art, as well as traditional modes of inquiry, as valued methods in the search for meaning in the lived experience (Giorgi, 1970). We need to seek new ways of being and knowing, alternatives to the routine (Greene, 1988). Watson (1988) encouraged us to try a new language, a new metaphor, in order to capture "unique notions" about the nature of the human being, the human center, and "the human dimensions that occur in the lived moment . . . of human caring" (p. 177). Aesthetics and intuitive modes of awareness offer precognitive insights into the nature of our being and the meaning of our being-in-this-world. Creativity and aesthetics have a "dual role. . . . [They] enlarge the universe by adding or uncovering new dimensions. [They] also enrich and expand man, who will be able to experience these new dimensions inwardly" (Arieti, 1976, p. 5). As such, aesthetics contribute to the process of healing and health promotion.

Two aesthetic modalities that are particularly useful as health promotion and healing techniques are photography and storytelling. Photographs serve as a reminder that an aspect has importance in life. They can be analyzed by the photographer for recurrent themes or as a method of identifying aspects of life that one finds particularly pleasurable and meaningful. Stories are constructed and moments revisited so that meaning is extracted through personal self-reflection. Understanding of the intricacies and multiplicities of life is enhanced, and the inherent holistic nature of the universe is embraced and celebrated. Healing occurs.

Photography

Photography can be used to narrow the *visual* horizon to a manageable scope and to quiet the inner world of experience. Simultaneously, the *inner* horizon expands and diversifies, gaining significantly in the search for meaning and understanding of the human experience. The camera is used to capture the world that speaks to the inner self, the experiences as lived and cherished, those substances of existence with which we connect.

Photography has been widely used as a method of study in the social sciences and ethnography.

> *We play at social science. In "capturing the world" we test our ideas about each other against the photographs and the realities they represent. In "creating visual statements" we manifest our understanding of the interesting and important. Through the photographs we increase our knowledge of each other while at the same time raise questions about how well we understand our own lives. Through taking photographs . . . we participate in . . . scientific inquiry. (Wagner, 1979, p. 12)*

The camera as a research tool is a "legitimate abstracting process in observation" (Heider, 1972, p. 5). It helps to organize and refine the data collected, as it records a representation of the observed (Heider, 1972).

Are photographs mere images of truth and reality, or do they reflect the mind's-eye perspective of the photographer? Weston (1979) denounced "the folly of using a camera to imitate" the work of a painter and emphasized the need to "see photographically." Photography should be used to "heighten the sense of reality," revealing the "vital essences" of images as perceived by the photographer (Weston, 1979). The photographer *selects* the article photographed because it can "best express what it is we have to say" (Weston, 1979).

The person behind the lens shapes the reality photographed rather than being shaped by the objectiveness of the environment. Within the art of photography, the subjective multiplicities of reality come to life. Real harm lies in the beholdenness to reproduce "perfection" in photography. Rules regarding the management of equipment, correct composition, and lighting regulations stifle the artistic and creative values of seeing photographically. "By varying the position of his camera, his . . . angle, or the focal length of the lens, the photographer can achieve an infinite number of . . . compositions . . ." (Weston, 1979, p. 209). Therefore, reality is not recreated by the camera but created within the photographer.

The process of photography must be "regarded from onset as a whole" (Weston, 1979, p. 209). Lighting, color values, and strength of subject will become an intuitive process to create that piece of the world that the photographer perceives to be significant. Creation will also be intuitively harmonious with the image as it is perceived. Photographic seeing "searches out the actor behind the makeup and exposes the contrived, the trivial, the artificial, for what they really are. . . . It is basically too honest a medium for recording superficial aspects of a subject" (Weston, 1979, p. 210).

Therefore, photography is a legitimate method of personal inquiry, self-knowing, and health promotion. The self perceives aspects of the world to be energy-giving rather than energy-draining, and these aspects are then created in the photographic process and recorded by the medium. Through creative processes, the photographer, as a participant–observer in the ethnography of self, records the world of the self. Interpretation of the meaning of this world can then be attempted through studying this "seeing photograph" via a process of self-reflection, journaling, and storytelling. Just as the social scientist/ethnographer verifies the content of a photograph with a study participant, so may a photograph be explored by the photographer for inner meaning of self.

Storytelling

Coming to know the nature of personal reality, discovering the meaning of individual experience, and having glimpses into the nature of the implicate order of the whole are made possible through the process of storytelling. Storytelling, the aesthetic methodology of reflection, brings to consciousness those aspects of a person that are central to the nature of the human core and give purpose to existence (Malkani, 1966). Although this "knowledge" is not objectively verifiable, human beings use it to act on their reality; it is that which is considered to be important to self (Giorgi, 1970).

"Seeing photographically" necessitates self-reflection. The individual must reflect on the nature of the reality perceived and photographed, determining its importance and meaning in experiences as they are lived. Meaning and understanding in the phenomenological sense are gained through intensive interview with the individual and reflection on the words, text, and meaning within the lived experience, as described by the experiencing person (Merleau-Ponty, 1964). When studying the meaning of self and one's own lived experience, the individual uses the method of intensive self-reflection/self-interview and storytelling as a means of accessing intuitive awareness.

The self in dialogue is recorded in intensive journaling. The journal can then later be reviewed for achievement of thematic discovery, pattern recognition, and story development; the process is similar to phenomenological and ethnographic discovery. The emergence of themes and story lines assists the person in identifying new interpretations of information and facilitates healing as underlying, intersubjective, personal knowledge unfolds from the journaling process. The self is recognized and celebrated as connections move from precognitive to cognitive and creative awareness.

Additional information and pattern recognition can be gained by examining the photographs and journaling entries for similarities and contrasts. Impressively clear images often emerge during the comparative process, which lends insight into the nature of the relationships of self to the underlying order of the whole. The points of convergence between the aesthetic and personal modes of inquiry provide strong messages as to the nature of the mystical implicate order, inherently unknowable in totality (Bohm, 1980). Uncovering the "true reality . . . is not perceived by the senses" as if "separate from man" (Bohm, 1980, pp. 24–25). Rather, humans must give their full attention to creative energies that see the immeasurable in the illusion of self (Bohm, 1980).

Photography as described has been used in the search for health and healing. Individuals are able to employ the method through facilitation by nurse healers, who act as celebrants of the life processes, attending to the needs of persons in search of healing through transpersonal caring. Nurses in this type of practice do not attempt to lead the patient to right answers or correct behaviors. Rather, the nurses nurture the patients in their journey of self-discovery and illuminate meaning through caring presence. Aesthetic healing modalities of photography and storytelling can be used individually by any person acting as a participant–observer in the ethnography of self.

CONCLUSION

Life is a matter of becoming, a process of continual self-transformation and transcendence. To promote health and healing, individuals must be able to examine the nature of the self in relationship with the nature of the unitary order, the whole. Connections and purpose need to be ensured, realized, and illuminated. The innate God-in-me must be celebrated. This knowing–understanding is facilitated by becoming aware of the innate nature of the self as the seat of the soul and a reflection of the unitary consciousness. Human consciousness is expanded through the use of multiple modes of awareness which include aesthetics and personal knowing.

The nature of reflective storytelling and "photographically seeing" permits the unfolding of human purpose. Acknowledgement of self and its reflective nature reveals a personal knowledge that encourages humans to realize the unitary nature of their being, thus healing self. This empowering modality of healing permits the recipient to heal the I/me schism, enhancing a personal sense of well-being and becoming, and enabling human transcendence to what is not-yet.

REFERENCES

American heritage dictionary. (1980). Boston: Houghton-Mifflin.

Arieti, S. (1976). *Creativity: The magic synthesis.* New York: Basic Books.

Bach, R. (1977). *Illusions: The adventures of a reluctant messiah.* New York: Dell.

Bach, R. (1988). *One.* New York: Dell.

Baumann, A., & Deber, R. (1989). The limits of decision analysis for rapid decision making in ICU nursing. *Image: The Journal of Nursing Scholarship, 21*(2), 69-71.

Benner, P. (1984). *From novice to expert: Excellence and power in clinical nursing practice.* Menlo Park, CA: Addison-Wesley.

Bohm, D. (1980). *Wholeness and the implicate order.* London: Routledge & Kegan Paul.

Bohm, D. (1985). *Unfolding meaning.* London: Ark Paperbacks.

Bohm, D. (1987). *Science, order, and creativity.* Toronto, Canada: Bantam Books.

Carper, B. (1978). Fundamental patterns of knowing in nursing. *Advances in Nursing Science, 1*(1), 13-23.

Center for Disease Control. (1992). *Morbidity and mortality: 1991.* Atlanta, GA: The Center.

Giorgi, A. (1970). *Psychology as a human science.* New York: Harper & Row.

Greene, M. (1988). *The dialectic of freedom.* New York: Teachers College Press.

Grof, S. (1985). *Beyond the brain.* Albany: SUNY Press.

Grof, S. (1988a). *The adventure in self-discovery.* Albany: SUNY Press.

Grof, S. (Ed.). (1988b). *Human survival and consciousness evolution.* Albany: SUNY Press.

Grof, C., & Grof, S. (1990). *The stormy search for self.* Los Angeles: Tarcher.

Hammersly, M., & Atkinson, P. (1983). *Ethnography principles and practice.* London: Tavistock Publications.

Heider, C. (1972). *Film for anthropological teaching.* Philadelphia: Temple University Press.

Kafka, F. (1972). *The Metamorphosis.* Toronto: Bantam.

Keller, M. (1981). Toward a definition of health. *Advances in Nursing Science, 4*(1), 43-64.

Malkani, G. (1966). *Philosophy of the self.* New York: Johnson Reprint.

Meleis, A. (1991). *Theoretical nursing: Development and progress.* Philadelphia: Lippincott.

Merleau-Ponty, M. (1964). Phenomenology and the science of man. In Edie, J. (Ed.), *The Primacy of Perception.* Evanston: Northwestern University Press.

Newman, M. (1979). *Theory development in nursing.* Philadelphia: F. A. Davis.

Newman, M. (1986). *Health as expanding consciousness.* St. Louis: C. V. Mosby.

Newman, M. (1990). Shifting to higher consciousness. In M. Parker (Ed.), *Nursing theories in practice* (pp. 129-140). New York: National League for Nursing.

Newman, M., Sime, A., & Corcoran-Perry, S. (1991). The focus of the discipline of nursing. *Advances in Nursing, 14*(1), 1-14.

Parse, R. (1987). *Nursing science: Major paradigms, theories, and critiques.* Philadelphia: W.B. Saunders.

Parse, R. (1990a). Promotion and prevention: Two distinct cosmologies. *Nursing Science Quarterly, 3,* 101.

Parse, R. (1990b). Health: A Personal Commitment. *Nursing Science Quarterly, 3,* 136-140.

Parse, R. (1992). Human becoming: Parse's theory of nursing. *Nursing Science Quarterly, 5*(1), 35-42.

Polanyi, AM., & Prosch, H. (1975). *Meaning.* Chicago: University of Chicago Press.

Prabhavananda, S. (1948). *The Upanishads.* New York: Mentor Books.

Prescott, P., Dennis, K., & Jacox, A. (1987). Clinical decision making of staff nurses. *Image, 19*(2), 56-62.

Quinn, J. (1989). The Haelen effect. *Nursing and Health Care, 10*(10), 552-557.

Rew, L. (1988). Intuition in decision-making. *Image, 20*(3), 150-154.

Rogers, M. (1970). *The theoretical basis of nursing.* Philadelphia: F. A. Davis.

Rogers, M. (1986). Science of Unitary Human Beings. In V. Malinski (Ed.), *Explorations on Martha Rogers' Science of Unitary Human Beings* (pp. 3-14). Norwalk: Appleton-Century-Crofts.

Rogers, M. (1988). Nursing science and art: A prospective. *Nursing Science Quarterly, 1,* 99-102.

Rogers, M. (1990). Nursing: Science of unitary, irreducible, human beings: Update 1990. In E. Barrett (Ed.), *Visions of Rogers' science-based nursing* (pp. 5-12). New York: National League for Nursing.

Rogers, M. (1993, January). Personal interview. Phoenix, Arizona.

Smith, J. (1983). *The idea of health.* New York: Teachers College Press.

Smith, M. (1990). Nursing's unique focus on health promotion. *Nursing Science Quarterly, 3*(3), 105-106.

Wagner, J. (1979). *Images of information.* Beverly Hills: Sage University Press.

Watson, J. (1985a). *Nursing: Human science and human care.* Norwalk: Appleton-Century-Crofts.

Watson, J. (1985b). *Nursing: The philosophy and science of caring.* Boulder, CO: Associated University Press.

Watson, J. (1988). New dimensions of human caring theory. *Nursing Science Quarterly, 1*(3), 175-181.

Watson, J. (1989). Human caring and suffering: A subjective model for health science. In R. Taylor and J. Watson (Ed.), *They Shall not Hurt* (pp. 125-135). Boulder: University of Colorado Press.

Watson, J. (1990a). Caring knowledge and informed moral passion. *Advances in Nursing Science, 13*(1), 15-23.

Watson, J. (1990b). Transpersonal caring: A transcendent view of person, health, and healing. In M. Parker (Ed.), *Nursing theories in practice* (pp. 277-288). New York: National League for Nursing.

Watson, J. (1990c). The moral failure of the patriarchy. *Nursing Outlook, 38*(2), 62-66.

Watson, J. (1992, January). *Theory in human care nursing.* Symposium conducted at the University of Colorado Health Sciences Center, Boulder.

Watson, J. (1993, February). Personal interview. Las Vegas, NV/ Boulder, CO.

Weston, E. (1979). Seeing photographically. In M. Rader (Ed.), *A book of modern esthetics.* New York: Holt, Rinehart, and Winston.

13

Children's Drawings: A Different Window

Judy Malkiewicz
Marilyn L. Stember

*A*lthough the use of children's art in nursing has expanded in recent decades, nurses are not well prepared to understand these artistic expressions. This chapter makes explicit the potential contributions and challenges of children's drawings and suggests issues to consider in using art in nursing practice and research.

Children's drawings have been successfully used by health and educational professionals as assessment, diagnostic, and psychoanalytic tools (Anastasi, 1976; Burgess, McCausland & Wolbert, 1981; Handler & Reyher, 1966; Hibbard & Hartman, 1990; Hibbard, Roghmann, & Hoekelman, 1987; Impey, 1981; Kaufman & Wohl, 1992; Krahn, 1985; Perlman & Abramovitch, 1987; Petrie, 1954; Philipp, Philipp, Pendered, Barnard, & Hall, 1986; Spinetta

& Deasy-Spinetta, 1981; Spinetta, McLaren, Fox, & Sparta, 1981; Stember, 1980; Unruh, McGrath, Cunningham, & Humphrey, 1983; Yates, Beutler, & Crago, 1985; Zinsmeister, 1990). Others have used children's drawings to assess developmental aspects in children, including personality development, manual skills, cognitive development, maturity, and emotional status (e.g., Bender, 1952; DiLeo, 1973; Golumb, 1974; Goodenough, 1926; Harris, 1963; Koppitz, 1968; Machover, 1949).

Recognizing the utility of this medium, nursing has incorporated children's art as screening, therapeutic, and research tools (e.g., Gelhard, 1978; Johnson, 1990; Lynn, 1986, 1987; McLeavey, 1979; Poster, 1989). Nurses have used children's drawings to identify children's feelings about topics such as being hospitalized or going to the doctor's office (Allen, 1978; Baretich, Stephenson, & Igoe, 1989; Irwin & Kovacs, 1979; Jones & Wakeley, 1974; Malkiewicz & Stember, 1988; Nadler, 1983; Plonk, 1971; Romero, 1985; Shrewsbury, 1987; Stember, 1988; Vanek, 1979). Other nurses have used drawings to determine children's views of being physically, sexually, or emotionally abused (Burgess, 1988; Kelley, 1985; Malkiewicz, 1991; Scavnicky-Mylant, 1986) as well as to learn more about children's concepts of body image (Badger & Jones, 1990; Burns, Cameron, Juszczak, & Wallace, 1984; Johnson, 1990).

Art is increasingly considered by nursing theorists as an important element of nursing. Art was described by Watson (1985) as a human-to-human means of establishing relationships between nurses and the recipients of care, thus allowing the genuine transmission of feelings. Paterson and Zderad (1976) noted that "forms of art are valued as resources for enriching our knowledge of man and the human situation." Although children's drawings are intuitively appealing and easy to implement, nurses are not well-prepared to use these artistic expressions. This chapter identifies the vast potential and numerous challenges associated with using this art form and suggests issues to consider in using children's drawings in nursing practice and research.

In summarizing a century of children's drawings, Strommen (1988) pointed to the evolution of theory and research. Initially, human figure drawings and other drawings were used as projctive assessment tools for evaluating cognitive development and intelligence (Goodenough, 1926). Children's drawings also have been used to determine emotional indicators in children, as art has been thought to be an unconscious projection of self that is useful for identifying concerns and feelings (Koppitz, 1968; Oster & Gould, 1987). More recently, spontaneous and other expressive drawings have been used to gain insight into children's experiences and feelings. Figure 1, a 9-year-old boy's drawing about being disciplined, portrays his strong emotional response.

Drawing is a natural mode of expression for children. Many children who are incapable of conveying their feelings and attitudes through verbal or written communication may be able to express themselves through drawing (Koppitz, 1968). Young children are not always capable of verbalizing their experiences,

Figure 1. Nine-year-old boy: emotional response to parental discipline. "Well, my dad grabs his whip or his belt. I'm scared, man . . . to get my butt real sore . . . my butt's going to be real sore."

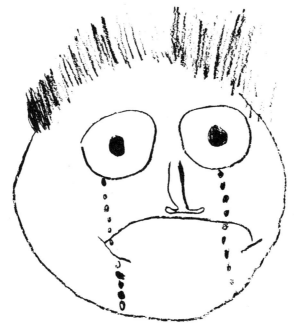

especially with an adult stranger. Using children's drawings to generate additional clinical or research data has great potential in nursing. Children older than 5 and younger than 12 years of age will usually produce and describe their drawings without much hesitation. Beyond 12, children are likely to refuse to draw unless they view themselves as artistic (Edwards, 1989). Hence, drawings are an important vehicle for preadolescent children to tell their stories, express their feelings, and work out their problems.

For users of drawings, the central concern is the validity of interpretations. Drawings are often under- or overinterpreted (Scavnicky-Mylant, 1986; Spinetta et al., 1981). Scoring schemes, although widely used, have not always held up well in validity and reliability studies (Falk, 1981; Lingren, 1971; Tharinger & Stark, 1990). Children's drawings show a marked developmental change over time, from preschematic to realistic (Gelhard, 1978; Groves & Fried, 1991; Lowenfeld & Brittain, 1966; Mitchelmore, 1978; Nicholls & Kennedy, 1992). Further complexities may be introduced by the influence of contextual events (Sturner, Rothbaum, Visintainer, & Wolfer, 1980) as well as the child's gender (Silk & Thomas, 1986). Even when children provide accompanying verbal explanations, they may not be able to corroborate the expressions apparent in their drawing; if the topic is too painful, a child may say the active person is another child with this problem. Further, subjective agreement or reliability is not easy to achieve. Thus, many issues must be considered in using artistic methods with children.

SELECTING A DRAWING EXPERIENCE

Most assessment techniques using children's drawings are projective. They include Draw-A-Person, Kinetic Family Drawing, House-Person-Tree, Draw-A-Situation, and other less frequently used techniques such as Drawing Completion, A Favorite Kind of Day, and Draw-A-Story (Neale & Rosal, 1993). Spontaneous drawings are also used as an alternative to these standardized tools.

Draw-A-Person

Developed by Goodenough (1926), the instructions for the Draw-A-Person assessment are to "draw a complete person." This human drawing tool is widely accepted as being the closest to a child's inner self-portrait. Drawing a person elicits feelings about self, personality traits, attitudes, concerns, and interpersonal skills. When analyzing these drawings, Wohl and Kaufman (1985) suggested: "[T]he examiner studies the drawing, noting the general themes of size, placement, line quality and pressure, spontaneity or rigidity, and the emotions it elicits. . . . Attention is then paid to the inclusion and omission of numerous specifics, such as the head, facial features, body and body parts, limbs, hands, fingers, clothing, and the presence of extraneous details, such as clouds or another person" (pp. 11-12). Although these human figure drawings are most often systematically scored (Engle & Suppes, 1970; Harris, 1963; Koppitz, 1966; Machover, 1967; Phillips & Smith, 1973; Simner, 1985), they also have been qualitatively analyzed using varying approaches.

The Draw-A-Person has been successfully used in nursing. Badger and Jones (1990), in their study of 80 deaf children and 190 normal-hearing children aged 5 to 15 years, found the Draw-A-Person test to be particularly useful because of its nonverbal, nonacoustic content and straightforward scoring procedure. In a study of 30 hospitalized children and 30 control children, Irwin and Kovacs (1979) found significant differences between pre- and postoperative pictures (e.g., exaggerated, reduced, or otherwise distorted proportions; certainty of stroke; stability; and pencil pressure). They concluded that findings from the drawings loosely paralleled the children's verbal stories.

Kinetic Family Drawing

In the Kinetic Family Drawing developed by Burns and Kaufman (1970), children are instructed to "draw your family doing something." This assessment examines the child's subjective family experience and view of family interactions (Burns, 1982). Some qualitative analysts of these family pictures ask themselves: What was my first impression? Whom and what did I see? What is happening? How do I feel about what is happening? Would I like to be a member of this family? In their qualitatively integrated system, Tharinger and Stark (1990) rated four characteristics on a five-point scale to gain a holistic sense of the family drawings. Others (e.g., Spinetta et al., 1981) have developed structured scoring procedures for this test. Whether qualitatively or quantitatively analyzed, these action drawings symbolize how certain family members are perceived by the child. Only a few studies in the nursing literature used family drawings. For example, Johnson (1990) analyzed family drawings using subjective and objective interpretations in four case studies.

House-Tree-Person

In another assessment technique, the House-Tree-Person drawing test (Buck, 1948; Hammer, 1958), four drawings are requested: (1) a house, (2) a tree, (3) a person, and (4) a person of the opposite sex. Symbolically, the house is purported to reflect the child's body image, maturity, adjustment, accessibility to others, contact with reality, and general emotional stability (Buck, 1981; Wohl & Kaufman, 1985). The house may also reveal the child's view of his or her home life, the quality of family relationships, and the child's attitudes toward parents and siblings (DiLeo, 1983; Wohl & Kaufman, 1985). The tree is thought to represent the life and growth of the personality. Elements of the personality are projected in the manner in which the child draws the tree. "By allowing ourselves to experience the total gestalt of the tree, without focusing on the details, we can understand the inner picture of the youngster's life" (Wohl & Kaufman, 1985, p. 114). More specifically, the tree trunk is thought to represent feelings of inner strength, and the branches are associated with the ability to derive satisfaction from the environment. In a nursing research study of children of alcoholics, Scavnicky-Mylant (1986) used the House-Tree-Person drawing test. She found that, although the children of alcoholics drew pictures of houses as directed, the house drawings were immature and most children refused to talk about them. In each of the house, person, and tree picture types, she found reflections of denial, poor self-image, powerlessness, and feelings of responsibility.

Draw-A-Situation

Most widely used in nursing, the Draw-A-Situation format permits the user to focus the child's attention on a particular topic or situation. For example, "What would it be like to be in a hospital?" (Allen, 1978) or "Draw a picture of what it is like to be disciplined by your parents" (Malkiewicz, 1991). This approach has the advantage of helping the child focus on a situation, providing the opportunity to obtain richer detail in the area of interest.

This technique, however, is not without difficulties. Some children will draw a "literal interpretation." Figure 2, drawn by a first-grade boy, is his response to the request to "Draw a picture of what happens when you go to see a doctor or school nurse" (Stember, 1988). Instead of depicting people and activities in the health provider's office, like most children, this young boy drew a picture of himself in the car literally *going* to the doctor's office.

Figure 2. First-grade boy's literal translation of *going* to doctor's office in a car.

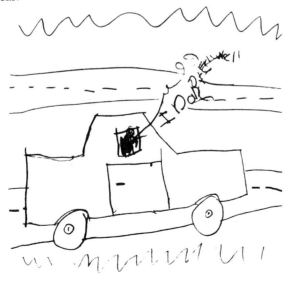

ESTABLISHING MEANING

Researchers and clinicians using children's drawings have applied a variety of methods for analyzing drawings. They have ranged from specific scoring schemes to global qualitative assessments. Various drawing indicators have been assessed and assigned meaning. For example, poor integration of parts in the Draw-A-Person or other human-figure drawings is associated with anxiety and impulsivity. Shading reflects anxiety; slanting figures reflect instability and mental imbalance; tiny figures reflect insecurity, withdrawal, depression, and feelings of inadequacy; big figures reflect security, relaxation, expansiveness, or poor inner controls; and omission of arms reflects guilt over hostility or sexuality (Baldwin, 1966; DiLeo, 1973; Hammer & Kaplan, 1966; Koppitz, 1966, 1968; Machover, 1949; Oster & Gould, 1987).

Horizontal orientations to pictures are associated with more passive children; vertical orientations are associated with more assertive children (Stember, 1980). Light, wavering, or broken lines are related to more insecure children; bold, continued, freely drawn lines indicate self-confidence (DiLeo, 1983; Koppitz, 1966, 1968). Omission and distortion of body parts often indicate anxiety (Handler & Reyher, 1966; Koppitz, 1966). Relative size, proximity, and facial expressions provide insights into the child's interpersonal relationships (Koppitz, 1968; Thomas & Gray, 1992).

Children will emphasize and exaggerate parts of the drawing considered most important or holding special meaning for the child (Fox & Thomas, 1990, Machover, 1949). Figure 3, drawn by a fourth-grade girl, clearly demonstrates her fear of injections (Stember, 1988). Allen (1978) found that "instruments, such as thermometers and syringes, were drawn hugely out of proportion, sometimes floating conspicuously in the air and other times inflicting pain in people" (p. 28).

To a limited extent, drawings have been used to examine children's relationship with the health care provider. Several studies in dental research have used drawings to measure children's response to dental visits, with and without previsit preparation (Baldwin, 1966; Eichenbaum & Dunn, 1971; Sheskin, Klein, & Lowenthal, 1982; Sonnenberg & Venham, 1977). Using size of

Figure 3. Fourth-grade girl's drawing of nurse with injection needle and child yelling for help.

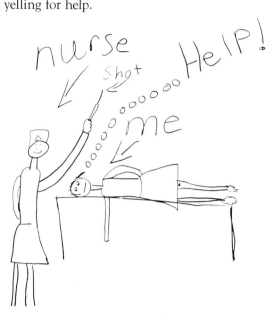

figures as the criterion, Baldwin (1966) demonstrated with serial human-figure drawings that children who were prepared for dental extraction recovered more rapidly than children who were not given prior preparation. Children were asked to draw four pictures: (1) baseline, before the first dental visit; (2) just prior to the dental extraction; (3) just after the extraction; and (4) several weeks after the extraction. Just prior to and just after extraction, children in both groups drew figures that were diminished in size from their baseline drawings. Children who had had dental extraction preparation, however, showed a statistically significant recovery in the size of their human-figure drawings following extraction. Children without dental extraction preparation continued to draw diminished human figures for up to a year following their extractions.

Although many investigators have used one or more dimensions and counted the occurrence, many proponents of human-figure drawing assessment tools suggest that no one-to-one relationship exists between a specific element of the drawing and a definite personality or emotional trait. Rather, the total drawing, in context with the specific information known about the child drawing the picture, should be considered in analyzing and interpreting the drawing (DiLeo, 1983; Koppitz, 1968, Machover, 1949; Oster & Gould, 1987). Further, regardless of the drawing tools used, children should, when possible, be encouraged to verbally explain their completed drawings. This explanation period may be expanded so that the clinician or researcher may ask for clarification of drawing elements not initially discussed. Wohl and Kaufman (1985) referred to this process as "post-drawing interrogation."

ELABORATING WITH ART

Although many earlier studies in nursing and other fields used children's art as the sole measurement of some phenomenon, the limitations of its singular use and its potential enhancing quality suggest using drawings as an adjunct with other clinical or research data. The authors' experience with two different research designs illustrates how drawings can be highly complementary to other research methods.

Malkiewicz (1991) studied the lived experience of parental discipline for 9- and 10-year-old children of middle-income families. In this phenomenologic hermeneutical study, 15 children were interviewed individually and in groups regarding their experience of being disciplined by their parent(s). Interviewing children can be a challenging endeavor. Building rapport with them is an important consideration: many children view discussions with adults as potentially threatening. Even when techniques such as asking simple versus complex questions (Barker, 1990) and reflecting the child's responses back to the child (Looff, 1976) were employed in this study, children had difficulty verbalizing. The times when these hesitations occurred were ideal for inviting the child to draw a picture of what it was like to be disciplined. This strategy was supported by van Manen (1984, 1990) and Chasin (1989), who suggested that the best way to elicit more detail is to ask children to draw a picture of the situation or experience of interest and have the children explain their drawings.

This combined methodology uncovered more of the participating children's lived experience associated with parental discipline (Malkiewicz, 1991). These 9- and 10-year-old children readily produced and described their drawings related to the discipline experience. Most children affirmed and added to their own and the investigator's understanding with their drawings and explanations.

Mad and sad feelings were by far the most common and most intensely stated emotions depicted in drawings of the parental discipline experience. Many children described their lived experience of parental discipline in metaphoric language as they drew and explained their drawings. This suggested the importance of using varied creative data-generation techniques with children. Metaphors of the lived experience of parental discipline included: mad as war (Figures 4 and 5), mad as a lion (Figure 6), mad as violent weather (Figure 7), sad as a basset hound (Figure 8), and sad as a broken heart (Figure 9).

The metaphors chosen by the children in the study both complemented and illuminated their experiences of parental discipline. Some drew themselves expressing an emotion such as mad, sad (Figure 10), afraid, and sorry. Others drew literal drawings of being spanked (Figure 11), yelled at, sitting alone in their room, or lying down. Other children drew fantasy thoughts: hitting a punching bag (Figure 12) or killing their parents (Figure 13).

Intensity of feelings related to the parental discipline experiences were especially vivid in the drawings of the children. For example, one 9-year-old girl drew an intense expression of her mad feelings when she depicted herself commanding a military tank blowing up her parents (Figure 4). As this young girl began to share the explanation of her picture, she crossed it out, turned her

Figure 4. Nine-year-old girl mad as war.

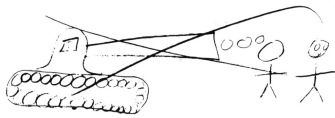

Figure 5. Same 9-year-old girl in second drawing of mad as war. "Well, sometimes, well, if your parents are kinda mean, sometimes you get mad at them and you don't want them to be alive and I don't think that but some kids might and so, I drew, drew like a cannon and then their parents are standing there. . . . Well, some people might think that, but they really don't mean it—but they are really mad at them."

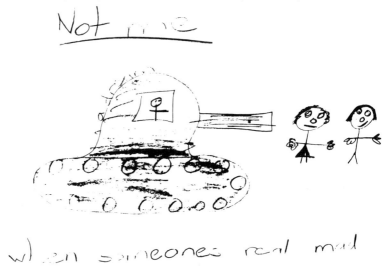

Figure 6. Nine-year-old girl mad as a lion. "That's suppose to be a lion, but I can't draw so. . . . That's suppose to be, ummm, a lion getting mad . . . or, like, a lion; you could just bite or roar or something . . . scream or something."

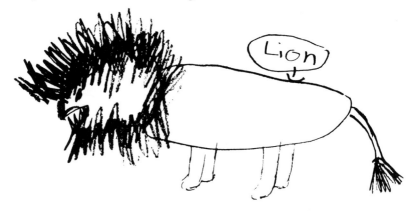

Figure 7. Nine-year-old boy disappointed. "This is a cloud and rainy and, humm, this means I'm unhappy. Unhappiness . . . cause, like, most people, like, well, like, they don't like rain because they, like, have a great day planned and something goes wrong and then it rains and you can't go on a picnic . . . it's disappointing . . . ."

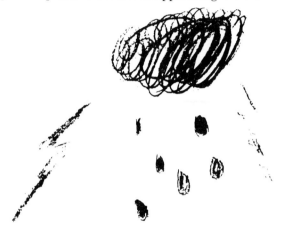

Figure 8. Nine-year-old girl sad like a basset hound. No verbal explanation given.

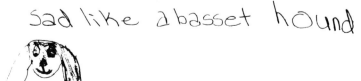

Figure 9. Nine-year-old girl with heart broken. "You sorta feel heart-broken when, humm, like, if you get yelled at or something . . . you don't feel very good and you feel heartbroken."

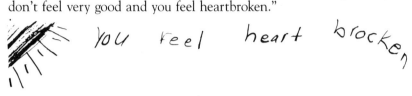

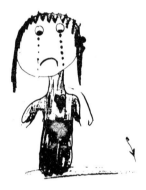

Figure 10. Nine-year-old girl sitting in room crying. "Well, it's just me sitting sad in my room mostly. These are my shelves. I'm trapped in my room . . . I don't have a door."

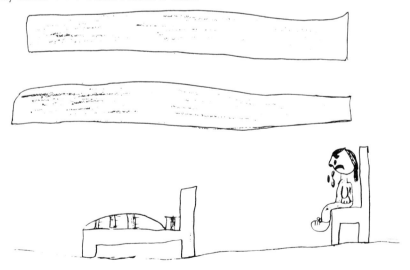

Figure 11. Nine-year-old boy being spanked. "Well, that's my dad with the paddle, that's my sister. My sister doesn't like me getting spanked and I'm crying."

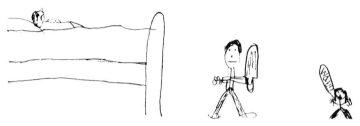

Figure 12. Nine-year-old boy with punching bag. "I feel like having a punching bag in my room and just hitting it really . . . Everlast, that's the name of the punching bag."

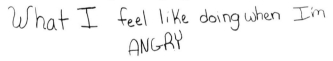

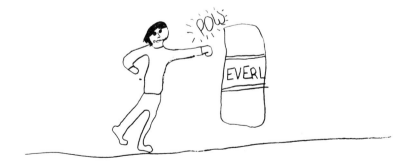

Figure 13. Nine-year-old boy with thoughts of killing parents. "Well, he's got a knife in the picture . . . okay . . . he's . . . I drew it when . . . sometimes when I get mad, err, disciplined, I feel like killing my parents. See there is me and there's the parent . . . and see I got the knife there. Well, it's not me but . . . could feel that bad."

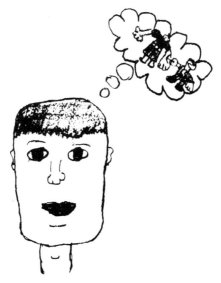

paper over, and drew the picture larger and with more detail, labeling it "a dream and when some other child is real mad" (Figure 5). She was more comfortable attributing the mad feelings to some other child, as revealed in the larger, more detailed second drawing. Without the drawings and their explanation, the researcher would not have realized the intensity of this little girl's mad feelings. In her verbal interview data, she matter-of-factly stated that she felt mad after her parents sent her to her room.

Stember's (1988) research on the effectiveness of HealthPACT is a second example of drawings to complement another primary study design. This experimental study of 946 children was conducted at seven elementary school sites in five states. Students in first, fourth, and sixth grades were randomly assigned to experimental and control groups. The intervention was HealthPACT, a health education program implemented in school settings and designed to teach children assertive and participatory health consumer behaviors and positive health habits. Outcome measures were obtained at baseline and at three posttest intervals approximately four months apart. At each measurement period, children were asked to draw a picture of what happened when they went to see a doctor or nurse.

To analyze these drawings, a new scoring scheme was derived from previous work in children's art. The Stember Artistic Reflection of Kids as Consumers (SARKC) Index initially included 21 dimensions (e.g., horizontal–vertical position, relative size of provider/child, omissions, interactive behavior). To evaluate the psychometrics of this scoring instrument, Malkiewicz and Stember (1988) conducted a reliability and validity study. The sample for this study was 216 children (72 from each of three grades, completely balanced for treatment and gender) who had participated in the larger experimental study and had completed all four drawings. These 826 drawings were independently evaluated by two raters, achieving an 85 percent interrater reliability. In refining the index, 15 items were retained, demonstrating very good construct validity and internal consistency reliability. Two subscales were identified (Anxiety and Participation) within the overall Consumerism Index, and these were found to have nearly adequate internal consistency reliability. Sensitivity to experimental treatment (HealthPACT) was demonstrated best after four months and decreased over eight to twelve months. A sequence of drawings from a fourth-grade girl reflects this increased participation (Figure 14(a)–(d)). Figure 14(a), a drawing completed at baseline, shows a passive horizontal posture. In Figure 14(b), drawn after implementing HealthPACT for one semester, this girl showed greater participation in the health visit, as illustrated by her sitting posture. In Figure 14(c), completed at the end of HealthPACT and the school year, she shows more active involvement and confidence in the health visit by her standing posture and hand position. Finally, in Figure 14(d), drawn after the summer vacation, this girl demonstrates less participation by her reclining posture. Another sequence of drawings from a sixth-grade girl (Figure 15(a)–(d)) illustrates a change in anxiety over time. The sequences were very similar to the results of the experimental study, which also showed some decline after the summer vacation.

Figure 14(a). At baseline, fourth-grade girl in passive, horizontal position.

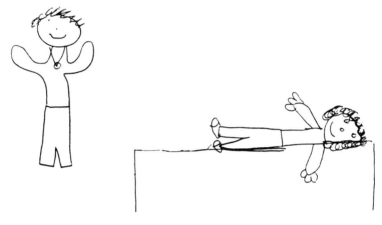

Figure 14(b). After one semester of HealthPACT program, same girl drew herself sitting up.

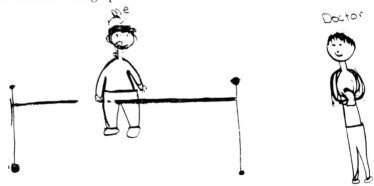

Figure 14(c). After two semesters of intervention, same girl appears more active.

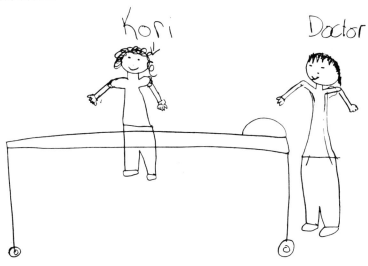

Figure 14(d). Drawn after summer vacation, same girl drew herself again in a more horizontal position.

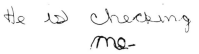

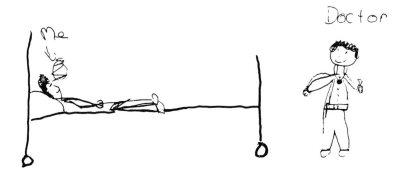

Figure 15(a). Sixth-grade girl expresses anxiety about visit to doctor's office (baseline).

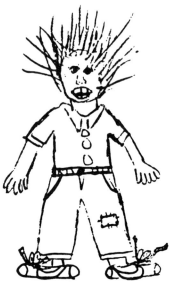

Figure 15(b). After one semester, hair and facial expression reflects less anxiety.

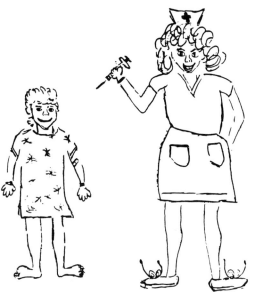

Figure 15(c). At end of intervention, same girl drew low anxiety and high participation.

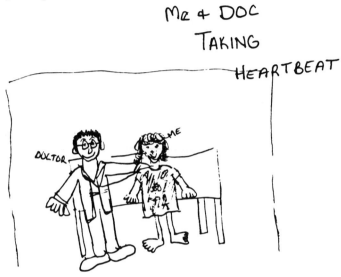

Figure 15(d). After summer vacation, same girl no longer smiling.

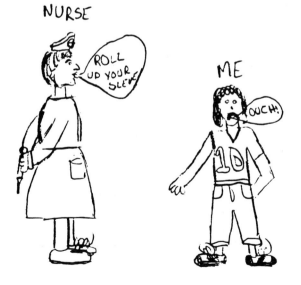

CONCLUSION

The art experience employs a creative process that integrates aesthetic, metaphorical, emotional, and physical dimensions. The emergent drawing is a concrete art form, an object in itself, with its own potentials. Not only can it be viewed for understanding, but it can also act as a stimulus for dialogue, thereby bridging past, present, and future understandings.

Drawings can be used in health care settings to open an avenue of communication with children, enabling nurses and other health care professionals to access more accurate and complete information. Although drawings may be difficult to evaluate, they may yield important additional knowledge about children, complementing other quantitative and qualitative data. Children's art provides a method of expression that verbal measures may not allow. Drawings may provide that different window needed for nursing's access into the child's world.

REFERENCES

Allen, J. M. (1978). Influencing school-age children's concept of hospitalization. *Pediatric Nursing, 4,* 26–28.

Anastasi, A. (1976). *Psychological testing* (4th ed.). New York: Macmillan.

Badger, T. A., & Jones, E. (1990). Deaf and hearing children's conceptions of the body interior. *Pediatric Nursing, 16*(2), 201–206.

Baldwin, D. C. (1966). An investigation of psychological and behavioral responses to dental extraction in children. *Journal of Dental Research, 45,* 1637–1651.

Baretich, D. M., Stephenson, P. A., & Igoe, J. B. (1989). Using art to understand children's perceptions of roles in physician's office visits. *Pediatric Nursing, 15*(4), 355–360.

Barker, P. (1990). *Clinical interviews with children and adolescents.* New York: Norton.

Bender, L. (1952). *Child psychiatric technique.* Springfield, IL: Thomas.

Buck, J. (1948). The house-tree-person technique: A qualitative scoring manual. *Journal of Clinical Psychology, 4*(4), 317–396.

Buck, J. (1981). *The House-Tree-Person technique.* Los Angeles: Western Psychologic Services.

Burgess, A. W., McCausland, M. P., & Wolbert, W. A. (1981). Children's drawings as indicators of sexual trauma. *Perspectives in Psychiatric Care, 19,* 50-58.

Burgess, E. J. (1988). Sexually abused children and their drawings. *Archives of Psychiatric Nursing, 2*(2), 65-73.

Burns, R. C. (1982). *Self-growth in families: Kinetic family drawing research and application.* New York: Brunner/Mazel.

Burns, R., Cameron, C. O., Juszczak, L., & Wallace, N. (1984). Using creative arts to help children cope with altered body image. *Journal of the Association for the Care of Children's Health, 12*(3), 108-112.

Burns, R. C., & Kaufman, S. H. (1970). *Kinetic family drawings: An introduction to understanding children through kinetic drawings.* New York: Brunner/Mazel.

Chasin, R. (1989). Interviewing families with children: Guidelines and suggestions. *Journal of Psychotherapy and the Family, 5*(3/4), 15-30.

DiLeo, J. H. (1973). *Children's drawings as diagnostic aids.* New York: Brunner/Mazel.

DiLeo, J. H. (1983). *Interpreting children's drawings.* New York: Brunner/Mazel.

Edwards, B. (1989). *Drawings on the right side of the brain: A course in enhancing creativity and artistic confidence* (rev. ed.). Los Angeles: Jeremy P. Tarcher.

Eichenbaum, I. W., & Dunn, N. A. (1971). Projective drawings by children under repeated dental stress. *Journal of Dentistry for Children, 38,* 169-170.

Engle, P. L., & Suppes, J. S. (1970). The relation between human figure drawing and test anxiety in children. *Journal of Projective Techniques and Personality Assessment, 34*(3), 223-231.

Falk, J. D. (1981). Understanding children's art: An analysis of the literature. *Journal of Personality Assessment, 45*(5), 465-472.

Fox, T. J., & Thomas, G. V. (1990). Children's drawings of an anxiety-eliciting topic: Effects on the size of the drawing. *British Journal of Clinical Psychology, 29,* 71-81.

Gelhard, H. L. (1978). Drawings and development. *Pediatric Nursing, 4,* 23-25.

Golumb, C. (1974). *Young children's sculpture and drawings.* Cambridge, MA: Harvard University Press.

Goodenough, F. (1926). *Measurement of intelligence by drawings.* New York: Harcourt, Brace & World.

Groves, J. R., & Fried, P. A. (1991). Developmental items on children's human figure drawings: A replication and extension of Koppitz to younger children. *Journal of Clinical Psychology, 47*(1), 140-148.

Hammer, M. (1958). *The clinical application of projective drawings.* Springfield, IL: Thomas.

Hammer, M., & Kaplan, A. M. (1964). The reliability of sex of first figure drawn by children. *Journal of Clinical Psychology, 20,* 251-252.

Hammer, M., & Kaplan, A. M. (1966). The reliability of children's human figure drawings. *Journal of Clinical Psychology, 22,* 316-319.

Handler, L., & Reyher, J. (1966). The relationship between GSR and anxiety indexes in projective drawings. *Journal of Consulting Psychology, 30*(1), 60-67.

Harris, D. B. (1963). *Children's drawings as measures of intellectual maturity.* New York: Harcourt, Brace & World.

Hibbard, R. A., & Hartman, G. L. (1990). Emotional indicators in human figure drawings of sexually victimized and nonabused children. *Journal of Clinical Psychology, 46*(2), 211-219.

Hibbard, R. A., Roghmann, K., & Hoekelman, R. A. (1987). Genitalia in children's drawings: An association with sexual abuse. *Pediatrics, 79*(1), 129-137.

Impey, L. (1981). Art media: A means to therapeutic communication with families. *Perspectives in Psychiatric Care, 19*(2), 70-77.

Irwin, E. C., & Kovacs, A. (1979). Analysis of children's drawings and stories. *Journal of the Association for the Care of Children's Health, 8*(2), 39-48.

Johnson, B. H. (1990). Children's drawings as a projective technique. *Pediatric Nursing, 16*(1), 11-17.

Jones, L., & Wakeley, C. (1974). Tell me about your picture: Insights into children's ideas about the hospital. *Imprint, 21,* 20-22, 29.

Kaufman, B., & Wohl, A. (1992). *Casualties of childhood: A development perspective on sexual abuse using projective drawings.* New York: Brunner/Mazel.

Kelley, S. J. (1985). Drawings: Critical communications for sexually abused children. *Pediatric Nursing, 11,* 421-426.

Koppitz, E. M. (1966). Emotional indicators on human figure drawings of children: A validation study. *Journal of Clinical Psychology, 22,* 313-315.

Koppitz, E. M. (1968). *Psychological evaluation of children's human figure drawings.* New York: Grune & Stratton.

Krahn, G. L. (1985). The use of projective assessment techniques in pediatric settings. *Journal of Pediatric Psychology, 10*(2), 179-193.

Lingren, R. H. (1971). An attempted replication of emotional indicators in human drawings by shy and aggressive children. *Psychological Reports, 29,* 35-38.

Looff, D. H. (1976). *Getting to know the troubled child.* Knoxville, TN: University of Tennessee Press.

Lowenfeld, V., & Brittain, W. L. (1966). *Creative and mental growth* (4th ed.). New York: Macmillan.

Lynn, M. R. (1986). Projective technique: A way of getting "hidden" information: Part I. *Journal of Pediatric Nursing, 1*(6), 407-408.

Lynn, M. R. (1987). Projective techniques in research and practice. *Journal of Pediatric Nursing, 2*(2), 129-131.

Machover, K. (1949). *Personality projection in the drawing of the human figure: A method of personality investigation* (10th ed.). Springfield, IL: Thomas.

Machover, K. (1967). *Personality projection in the drawings of the human figure.* Springfield, IL: Thomas.

Malkiewicz, J. (1991). Children's experience of parental discipline: A picnic spoiled. *Dissertation Abstracts International.* (University Microfilms No. 92-00,588 (DAO 72699).)

Malkiewicz, J., & Stember, M. (1988). *Estimates of psychometric properties of Stember's Artistic Reflection of Kids as Consumers Index.* Unpublished manuscript, University of Colorado Health Sciences Center, Denver.

McLeavey, K. A. (1979). Children's art as an assessment tool. *Pediatric Nursing, 5,* 9-14.

Mitchelmore, M. C. (1978). Developmental stages in children's representation of regular solid figures. *The Journal of Genetic Psychology, 133,* 229-239.

Nadler, H. S. (1983). Art experience and hospitalized children. *Children's Health Care, 11*(4), 160-164.

Neale, E. L., & Rosal, M. L. (1993). What can art therapists learn from the research on projective drawing techniques for children? A review of the literature. *The Arts in Psychotherapy, 20,* 37-49.

Nicholls, A. L., & Kennedy, J. M. (1992). Drawing development: From similarity of features to direction. *Child Development, 63,* 227-241.

Oster, G. D., & Gould, P. (1987). *Using drawings in assessment and therapy: A guide for mental health professionals.* New York: Brunner/Mazel.

Paterson, J., & Zderad, L. (1976). *Humanistic nursing.* New York: John Wiley & Sons.

Perlman, N., & Abramovitch, R. (1987). Clinical and laboratory observations: Visit to the pediatrician: Children's concerns. *Journal of Pediatrics, 110* (6), 988-990.

Petrie, M. (1954). *Art and regeneration.* London: Paul Elek.

Philipp, R., Philipp, E., Pendered, L., Barnard, C., & Hall, M. (1986). Can children's paintings of their doctors be interpreted? *Journal of the Royal College of General Practitioners, 36,* 325-327.

Phillips, C. J., & Smith, B. (1973). The Draw-A-Man test: A study of scoring methods, validity and norms with English children at five and eleven years. *Journal of Child Psychology and Psychiatry, 14,* 123-135.

Plonk, E. N. (1971). Working with children in hospitals (2nd ed.). Chicago: Case Western Reserve University Press.

Poster, E. C. (1989). The use of projective assessment techniques in pediatric research. *Journal of Pediatric Nursing, 4*(1), 26-35.

Romero, R. M. (1985). *Hospitalization as a life experience of the school-age child: An autobiographical journey.* Unpublished master's thesis, University of Colorado Health Sciences Center, Denver.

Scavnicky-Mylant, M. (1986). The use of drawings in the assessment and treatment of children of alcoholics. *Journal of Pediatric Nursing, 1*(3), 178-194.

Sheskin, R. B., Klein, H., & Lowenthal, V. (1982). Assessment of children's anxiety, throughout dental treatment, by their drawings. *Journal of Dentistry for Children, 49*(2), 99-106.

Shrewsbury, J. (1987). Painting: A coping device for preschool children. *Maternal-Child Nursing Journal, 11,* 11-16.

Silk, A. M. J., & Thomas, G. V. (1986). Development and differentiation in children's figure drawings. *British Journal of Psychology, 77,* 399-410.

Simner, M. L. (1985). School readiness and the Draw-A-Man test: An empirically derived alternative to Harris's scoring system. *Journal of Learning Disabilities, 18*(2), 77-82.

Sonnenberg, E., & Venhan, L. (1977). Human figure drawings as a measure of the child's response to dental visits. *Journal of Dentistry for Children, 44,* 438-442.

Spinetta, J. J., & Deasy-Spinetta, P. (Eds.). (1981). *Living with childhood cancer.* St. Louis: Mosby.

Spinetta, J. J., McLaren, H. H., Fox, R. W., & Sparta, S. N. (1981). The kinetic family drawing in childhood cancer: A revised application of an age-independent measure. In J. J. Spinetta & P. Deasy-Spinetta (Eds.), *Living with childhood cancer.* St. Louis: Mosby.

Stember, C. J. (1980). Art therapy: A new use in the diagnosis and treatment of sexually abused children. In B. Jones, L. Jenstrom, & K. MacFarlane (Eds.), *Sexual abuse of children: Selected readings* (DHHS Publication No. 59-63). Washington, DC: U.S. Government Printing Office.

Stember, M. L. (1988). *Kids as consumers: Effectiveness of HealthPACT* (Final report of "A study of school nurses' use of Project HealthPACT," U.S. Public Health Service Grant No. RO1 NU00993). Denver: University of Colorado Health Sciences Center.

Strommen, E. (1988). A century of children drawing: The evolution of theory and research concerning the drawings of children. *Visual Arts Research, 14*(2), 13-24.

Sturner, R. A., Rothbaum, F., Visintainer, M., & Wolfer, J. (1980). The effects of stress on children's human figure drawings. *Journal of Clinical Psychology, 36*(1), 324-331.

Tharinger, D. J., & Stark, K. (1990). A qualitative versus quantitative approach to evaluating the Draw-A-Person and Kinetic Family Drawing: A study of mood- and anxiety-disorder children. *Psychological Assessment, 2*(4), 365.

Thomas, G. V., & Gray, R. (1992). Children's drawings of topics differing in emotional significance—effects on placement relative to a self-drawing: A research note. *Journal of Child Psychology and Psychiatry, 33*(6), 1097-1104.

Unruh, A., McGrath, P., Cunningham, S. J., & Humphrey, P. (1983). Children's drawings of their pain. *Pain, 17,* 385-392.

Vanek, C. W. (1979). How school-age children perceive the intensive care unit environment. *Journal of the New York Student Nurses' Association, 10*(4), 30-34.

van Manen, M. (1984). Practicing phenomenological writing. *Phenomenology and pedagogy, 2*(1), 36-39.

van Manen, M. (1990). *Researching lived experience: Human science for an action-sensitive pedagogy.* Ann Arbor, MI: Althouse Press.

Watson, J. (1985). *Nursing: Human science and human care: A theory of nursing.* Norwalk, CT: Appleton-Century-Crofts.

Wohl, A., & Kaufman, B. (1985). *Silent screams and hidden cries: An interpretation of artwork by children from violent homes.* New York: Brunner/Mazel.

Yates, A., Beutler, L. E., & Crago, M. (1985). Drawings by child victims of incest. *Child Abuse & Neglect, 9,* 183-189.

Zinsmeister, K. (1990, June). Growing up scared. *The Almanac Monthly,* 49-66.

14

Aesthetic, Spiritual, Healing Dimensions in Music

Phyllis A. Updike

There will come a time when a diseased condition of the soul life will not be described as it is today by psychologists, but will be spoken of in musical terms, as one would speak, for instance, of a piano that was out of tune.

Rudolph Steiner

*T*raditionally, aesthetics as a branch of philosophy refers to the nature of the beautiful and judgments concerning beauty. However, the derivation from the Greek *aisthetikos* means sense perception. The French derivation from *aisthanesthai* means to perceive, with emphasis on the audible. These latter descriptors are particularly relevant to the perspective of this chapter.

Expressive feeling and *significant form* are two qualities shared by all good works of art. Feeling may be conceived as everything that can be felt and is not relegated to an emotional state exclusively. Feeling may be physical sensation, comfort, pain, excitement, reverie. A life that is *consciously* lived will allow for these sense perceptions. Langer (1976) proposed that music serves as a vehicle of feeling but not the individual feeling itself. Unique to music, in contrast to other classic art forms, is that it is suspended in the fourth dimension of time–space and is consequently the most abstract of structures. This means that, although not formless, its structure permits the individual maximum engagement: projection of his or her own unique experience free of external artistic definition of that subjective experience. In other words, a particular musical passage, or even an environmental sound, may be essentially one of joy, rage, sadness, triumph, or anguish, but it is free of any obligatory response by the listener. In other words, there is no specific artistic message that the listener is supposed to "get" or otherwise will have missed the message.

Significant form may be a familiar artistic structure such as a sonnet, ballad, classical ballet, madrigal, or symphony. On a wider scale, form may refer to the shape of a thing and/or a whole resulting from related mutually dependent factors. Abstract meaning is another expression of form. The bridge between Langer's conceptual work and relevance to human life and care of that life is not as illusive as it may appear. The shape of a thing in art may be compared to the shape or contour of a life—the rhythm, pulse, peaks, and troughs that characterize any consciously lived human life. The shape of a life in the midst of or subsequent to an illness or injury provides an intricate redefinition of that contour.

Creation of meaning of a musical selection is in the mind and imagination of the person. Creation of subjective meaning is now being lauded as a useful complementary healing modality; for example, a self-agency for adaptation and coping during an illness. In other words, subjective creation of the meaning of such an experience stands in equal stature with other more traditional coping mechanisms. Is this not the process of creating significant form to one's human condition? It becomes a way of creating connectedness among, at times, apparently fragmented and broken discontinuities. The aesthetic, sense-filled experience of music making and/or music listening may create a connection across the gap.

Manfred Clynes, an internationally acclaimed concert pianist and neuroscientist, has proposed that "music can engender the emotions as powerfully as a physical touch" (Clynes, 1982). The images and concretization of musical experience touching the feeling state and the body physical simultaneously, as expressed by an artist/scientist, is exciting and pertinent. Clynes has achieved critical pioneering work in articulating the nature of emotional responsiveness to music and how the conscious mind dynamically affects the physical body. He has outlined the neurobiologic process of recognition of pure emotion and how it may release in the brain specific substances that act to transmit and activate specific emotional experiences. This, in turn, may affect the autonomic and chemical process involved with hormonal mediation and short-term memory. The idea here is to perceive correlational, synchronous events rather than causative ones.

The speculated link between the language of music and neurobiologic properties is created by pulse and rhythm. According to Clynes, sentic (a biologically endowed form basic to expressive acts) forms denote emotional states and are represented primarily by anger, love, sex, grief, hate, joy, reverie. These emotional states appear to be genetically preserved forms of expressions. Another image of bridging, then, is that music moves—it is dynamic as it traverses time and space. The body–mind also moves, and it is also expressive. The movement, then, is embodied, both in music and in human form.

Dionysian and Apollonian modes of human experience further underline the aesthetic complement among art, music, and human processing (Clynes, 1980). The Dionysian mode implies potential physical responsiveness influenced by accompanying emotional patterns. Involvement of the whole body is emphasized here and this may be a mode we share with animal life.

The Apollonian mode involves a process of familiarity and recognition. The quality of the experience is contemplated or savored. This mode is particularly relevant to music, art, and aesthetic experience. It apparently is related to the way in which one experiences a flower—as "otherness."

In her recent book, *Composing a Life,* Mary Catherine Bateson (1990) discussed the importance of weaving, throughout one's life, a theme(s) that would serve to connect apparent discontinuities or fragmentation in human experience. She contended that the multiple interruptions—the hiccups—in one's life may actually be more interrelated than is apparent at first glance. She also believed that an aesthetic approach is requisite to success. She painted a large brush stroke to a frequently diminished sense of what is actually aesthetic:

> *Our aesthetic sense, whether in works of art or in our lives, has overly focused on a stubborn struggle toward a single goal rather than on fluid, protean, the improvisatory. (Bateson, 1990, p. 4)*

Composing a life has a metaphorical relationship to composing a work of art, for the life *can be* a work of art. Music making as a temporal art is a nonlinear (although sequential) pattern of audible diversity that transforms seeming fragmentation and chaos into a discernible pattern or configuration. Music embraces varied intensity, tempi, and rhythm. Life, consciously lived, embraces choices, rhythm, and a tempo that varies over time. Music listening, after critical selection, provides a sensate, perceivable vehicle that may foster the human dilemma of organizing a discontinuity of events. After all, learning from our interruptions may be very useful. It also provides the opportunity for one to become more fluid experientially.

What event precipitates a more profound, at times disturbing and abrupt, interruption than unexpected trauma or illness? Medications and treatment protocols may indeed have an effect on the problem, but may or may not heal the life. The process of improvisation is truly the means by which commitments are redefined and refocused—sometimes, but only sometimes, by choice. One of the most intriguing notions involves improvisation, time, and space:

> *If a unit of survival is an individual adapting to illness and recovery—If unit of survival is individual PLUS its environment, then sensitivity to environment is the highest of survival skills, not a dangerous distraction. We must live*

in a wider space and a longer stretch of time. (Bateson, 1990, p. 234)

Learning to live with a high degree of ambiguity is a valuable characteristic of an artist and manifests itself in art. Ambiguity is also implicit in living with paradox, which is characteristic of persons who have achieved a high level of moral/cognitive development. One might say that such persons have achieved artistry in living.

Viewing the body as music is not only an aesthetic reality but a psychophysiologic one. We know that the human body is very sensitive to perceived sound. Noise pollution has been named the most common modern health hazard (Dossey, 1992).

Noxious acoustical stimuli may be not only antithetical to the aesthetic, but may also trigger negative mind–body effects. Tachycardia, vasoconstriction, increased blood pressure, changed respiratory rate, and a shift in plasma cholesterol levels have been observed in response to noxious and/or high-volume sound environments. Although harmonic dissonance is disturbing, it seems that complete silence may be even more disturbing to some persons. It may be speculated that if the body demonstrates such specific physical reactivity, then the body itself could be said to have characteristics inherent in music itself. That is, the capacity to demonstrate movement in dimensions of time and space. If the body can respond so decisively to music, it must in some sense be music.

In *Nada-Brahma: The World Is Sound* (1987), musicologist Joachim-Ernst Berendt reminded us that the Latin term for "to sound through something" is *personare*. At the basis of concept of person stands concept of sound: "through the tone." If nothing sounds through from the bottom of the being, a human being is human biologically, at best, but is not a *per-son* because he or she does not live through the *son* (the tone, the sound). He or she does not live the sound which is the world (Berendt, 1987, p. 171).

In aboriginal legend, the world was sung into creation. Ritual use of chants, prayers, and incantations is truly worldwide. Certain sounds may well affect both physical *and* spiritual well-being, especially if we subscribe to the notion of embodied spirit.

Repetitive sound coupled with ritual techniques, plus expectation of intervention of God or the supernatural, allows other psychic or logical phenomena to unfold. Physically, repetitive auditory sound has a regulating effect on functioning. The future of music in physical therapy is very promising (Acterberg, 1992).

To recognize human psychophysiologic and psychospiritual challenges means to assess problems as well as gifts. New models of health and healing for individuals and communities for the 21st century are articulating this specific redefinition of assessment. Addressing risks and resiliencies affords new dimensions of effectiveness and inspiration. The intersection between this concept and the arts is that some human truths seem to be held only in the arts. Critical selection and intentional use of music listening can provide aesthetic and beneficial effects for the body–mind. This is a concrete example wherein the advancement of acoustic science will embrace the aesthetic potential.

The effectiveness of critically chosen music listening for enhanced well-being and function in humans has been well-documented in the literature. Music listening can relieve psychic and physical pain and discomfort. Just as medication or treatment protocols may be prescribed for specific use, therapeutic use of music may be intentionally prescribed to elicit desirable effects on the body–mind. One advantage offered by this complementary healing modality is a potential cognitive and perceptive shift in the relationship of the ill person to the dis/ease. That is, the caring/healing benefit of changing from a perspective of "Cancer has David" to "David has cancer" promotes a radical shift in the person's capacity toward empowerment.

There may be an existential parallel between the dynamic tempo of music and the experienced acceleration or deceleration of time in the midst of dis/ease, injury, or trauma. The *Andante, Allegro,* or *Vivace* of musical tempi are not unlike the varied passage of time in the presence of health and illness. Watson described caring healing consciousness as being temporally and spatially extended (Watson, 1987). Probably no other art form affords this existential possibility with more immediacy than does music listening.

Healing of the person's life as a whole may be independent of the health of individual parts, which may be tenuous at best. It is impossible to overestimate the necessity for intentional critical choice of the sound and music utilized. This is the distinction between music therapy and therapeutic use of music to facilitate a caring/healing milieu. Any environment may be acoustically full. Our everyday environment may be filled with voices, dishes, traffic, TV, stereo, intercoms, machines, and traffic, to name only a few sources of sound. We know that noxious acoustic environments may negatively affect blood pressure, respiratory rate, gastric enzyme secretion, and catecholamine release *regardless* of our attention to these sensate exposures. Music in all forms is not necessarily therapeutic either. Characteristics of tempo, irregular rhythms (e.g., 7/12 versus 3/4 or 4/4 time), or unresolved harmonics can negatively alter body–mind responses, *regardless* of our attentiveness to these sensory events.

If we consider our human biology in terms of musical form rather than mechanical construction and our responsiveness to biologic challenges as a repertoire of improvisations, we may find that disease restricts our ability to improvise new solutions to challenges—in musical terms, it restricts our ability to improvise. As an example, persons with disease may perceive and respond to music differently than do healthy people. Specifically, patients with tachycardia have shown a poor sense of rhythm perception and synchronization (Aldridge, 1993, p. 17).

Alfred Tomatis, a gifted French otolaryngologist, contributed pioneering work to the enlarged comprehension of the capacity to listen and its relation to the whole of the person (Belk, 1992; Gilmor, 1989). In 1947, Tomatis was hired by the French government to administer hearing tests to airline company employees. Tomatis discovered that standard hearing tests were measuring *listening* in addition to *hearing.* He realized that hearing loss, especially in high frequencies, profoundly affected the brain and its function. He eventually formulated his theory that sound is the unique sense that gives continuity to our lives; it is the fundamental building block of learning and communication. Sound is then an indicator not only of human function but also of human aesthetic experience!

Tomatis also verified that the human ear is the first developed sense organ in fetal life. Even prior to the ears' development, the fetus is responsive to sounds through bone conduction or somatic vibrations. The significance of this capacity has aesthetic and scientific value. If hearing pathways remain open and problem-free, learning and language skills develop normally. This pioneering work alone could provide a rich foundation for the importance of creating an acoustically aesthetic milieu for humanity's youngest members. Understandably, Tomatis has been sometimes called the Einstein of sound. Chinn (1989) has pointed out the importance of seeing the world through a lens of wholeness and integration in a way that never disregards a dimension of experience. This relationship of hearing, listening, mood, communication, and brain function is a significant example of Chinn's thought.

From optimal acoustic and aesthetic conditions for prenatal and postnatal life, let us shift now to music for the dying. Therese Schroeder-Sheker (1993) is the leading proponent of music thanatology. The term thanatology is derived from the name of Thanatos, the Greek god of death, and music thanatology is concerned with addressing the complex needs of the dying by conscious, intentional use of sound/music. The notion is founded on the practices of the monks in Cluny, France, in the 11th century. Central to Clunaic spirituality was a belief that the experience of beauty is an essential human need. The orientation was that the cultivation of beauty was one way to encounter the face of the Divine. Specifically, the Clunaic monks had such a powerful commitment to music that, at all monasteries, the monks were divided into cantors (singers) and conversi (nonsingers). Devotion to musical expression was exemplified in elaborate celebrations of the Mass. Monastic medicine in this community involved care of the body and cure of the soul. Attention was focused on the emotional, mental, physical, and spiritual pain that might prevent someone from experiencing a blessed death.

At the monastic infirmary at Cluny were found specific narratives of musical methods in tending dying persons. Just as the Clunaic infirmary offered a sanctuary to bridge life and a conscious death, the current aim of musical thanatology is to provide an aesthetically comforting journey through the same process today.

The live music that Schroeder-Sheker and her colleagues choose is individually prescriptive for each person's dying time. The Chalice of Repose project is a clinical and educational project located in Missoula, Montana (Schroeder-Sheker, 1993). The specific offerings of its ritual are called sound anointings. A person's favorite music is not often helpful. There is a critical difference between music for the living and music for the dying. Music for the living is intended to engage us; music for the dying is intended to free us.

We have come full circle in exploring the aesthetic need for critical care of our acoustic environment in birthing, living, and dying journeys. We have also explored the benefit of intentionally using music/sound/silence in health, illness and dis/ease, and healing experiences.

A new knowledge base is evolving, founded on the critical use and application of music/sound to facilitate beneficial effects for the psyche and soma. In the future, sound may be used more often with emphasis on its evocative potential.

Aesthetics and art exist not exclusively to placate and comfort, but to evoke images, ideas, and feelings. There are levels of self that often remain dormant. New science can assist, but, more importantly, the contemporary and global convergence among art, aesthetics, science, and spirit will be enhanced by using musical forms and sonor reflections.

In summary, how is it that music helps? Two primary categories emerge as distinctive:

1. Musical form can be an asset existentially, experientially, and metaphorically (e.g., dis-ease as a piano out of tune);
2. Musical form may elicit a psychophysiologic state that is not spirit itself but invites the spiritual domain to be exquisitely present as a source of strength and healing.

Musical experience seems to rest itself between phenomenon and thought, to locate itself ineffably between matter and spirit.

Each of us is blessed or cursed with 168 hours in each week. As we experience temporal dimensions in being born and dying, in health and illness, in woundedness and healing, it seems that conscious inclusion of the temporal art of musicality can be an aesthetic, spiritual, and healing dimension of our humanity.

REFERENCES

Acterberg, J. (1992). Drumming, shamanic work and healing: Interview by Don G. Campbell. In E. Bevis (Ed.), *Music and miracles* (pp. 123-127). Wheaton, IL: Quest Books.

Aldridge, D. (1993). Music of the body: Music therapy in medical settings. *Advances: Journal of Mind-Body Health, 9*(1).

Bateson, M. C. (1990). *Composing a life*. New York: Penguin.

Belk, J. (1992). Tomatis method: Auditory retraining through music and listening. In *Music and miracles* (pp. 242-250). Wheaton, IL: Quest Books.

Berendt, J. E. (1987). *Nada-brahma: The world is sound.* Rochester, VT: Destiny Books.

Chinn, P. (1989). Nursing patterns of knowing and feminist thought. *Nursing and Health Care, 10*(2), 71-75.

Clynes, M. (1980). *Communication of emotion: Theory of sentics in emotion, theory, research, and experience* (pp. 271-300). In R. Plutchick & H. Kellerman (Eds.), *Touch of Emotions,* Vol. I, New York: Academic Press.

Clynes, M. (Ed.). (1982). *Sentics: The touch of emotions.* New York: Plenum Press.

Dossey, L. (1992). The body as music. In L. Dossey (Ed.), *Music and miracles.* Wheaton, IL: Quest Books.

Langer, S. (Ed.). (1976). *Philosophy in a new key: A study in the symbolism of reason, rite and art.* Cambridge, MA: Harvard University Press.

Schroeder-Sheker, T. (1993). Music for the dying: A personal account of new field of music thanatology, history, theories, and clinical narratives. In *Advances, Journal of Body-Mind HHL, 9*(1), pp. 36-98.

Watson, J. (1987). The dream curriculum. In *Patterns on nursing: Strategies planning for nursing education* (pp. 91-104). New York: National League for Nursing.

15

The Use of Dance/ Movement Therapy in Psychosocial Nursing

D. Ellen Boyle

In the beginning came the dance.

My interest in movement therapy began back on Fifth Hall (an inpatient acute-care psychiatric unit in a general hospital in central Maine) when I, a psychosocial nurse, first witnessed a group of clients moving together. It was an exercise class and not formal "dance/movement therapy" at all; yet something was happening there, something "alive" that was palpable. I saw a 95-year-old woman, carrying the diagnosis "major depression, severe," tap her feet to the music and smile. I had never seen her smile. I saw a 15-year-old boy, who had a woeful family history and a long list of psychiatric symptoms, moving with this 95-year-old woman. The differences between them didn't seem to matter—there was some connection, something enlivening going on there. I was intrigued, fascinated, drawn in. So began this dance to bridge the gap between what I had seen and felt and intuited in that room full of movers and a rational understanding of what was happening and why and how.

This chapter begins with the conviction that nursing needs to restore value to and expand artistic process within the discipline. For the past several decades, there has been a steady expansion of the scientific base of nursing practice. This is a necessary and exciting development, but nursing will have greater potential to meet the serious health challenges of the 21st century if we expand our capacity to creatively interweave science and art into nursing theory, research, and practice. One primary effort toward accomplishing this important goal involves increasing the value of artistic endeavor in nursing. This is not to argue for throwing the science out in favor of the art, but rather for validating the latter and finding ways to interweave the esthetic and the empirical way of knowing.

One way of going about this growth process is for nursing to explore the approaches to psychotherapy used in the creative arts modalities. The idea is to link a creative process model with the systematic nursing process approach that is our discipline's strength. Examining a creative process model is a particularly appropriate approach in the fields of child and adolescent nursing, because all children normally grow and develop through creative processes. Johnston's (1986) Model of Creative Causality serves as the overall framework for this chapter; dance/movement is the particular form of creative process being explored.

Dance/movement therapy (DMT) is "the psychotherapeutic use of movement as a process which furthers the emotional and physical integration of the individual" (Schmais, 1974); it is the embodied form of the creative process. Theory from the DMT field will be interwoven throughout the section on "Creative Nursing Intervention," later in the chapter. The use of DMT will then be applied to a problem of paramount concern to child and adolescent psychosocial nursing: childhood sexual abuse (CSA).

The population of adolescent females with a history of CSA was selected because of the unique contribution to healing that dance and movement therapy can make with this group. The clinical picture of an adolescent with history of CSA presents with problems in three main areas: (1) self-concept, (2) affect regulation, and (3) interdependence.

Self-concept, the composite of beliefs and feelings that one holds about oneself at a given time, is formed by internal perceptions and the perception of others' reactions (Roy, 1976). It includes both the physical self and the personal self.

The physical self, which includes body sensations and body image, is impacted in clients with CSA. The adolescent girl with a history of CSA has difficulty being "in" her body; her body image tends to be distorted, and different parts of the body may be given unusual importance and meaning (Finklehor, 1986). There can be misperceptions around body sensations. Thus, a critical, first-stage goal of DMT is to address this area.

The personal self, consisting of self-consistency, self-ideal, and moral-ethical-spiritual self (Roy, 1976), is also impacted in CSA. The traumatized adolescent can find it hard to separate self from the abuse experience and may have difficulties with sexual identity, self-forgiveness, a sense of stigmatization, and a sense of inefficacy (Finklehor, 1986). DMT promotes a redeveloped sense of self by clearly delineating, through movement experiences, what is me/not me. Through the creative process, the client also gains a sense of the possibility of further self-development.

The client with CSA often presents with problems in interpersonal relationships. There is a tendency to display: overidealization or denigration of significant others, sexual dysfunction, outbursts of rage, or overly compliant behavior. DMT theory holds that a person normally develops the capacity for mutually satisfying relationships through close body contact/rhythms (Kestenberg & Sossin, 1979); when these are disrupted, the capacity for satisfying reciprocity is thwarted. DMT seeks to rebuild that capacity.

Finally, the CSA adolescent often has difficulty with affect regulation. The DMT process offers the possibility of emotional release of pent-up emotions as well as the opportunity to integrate these experiences.

The clinical illustrations in this chapter are drawn from an inpatient group of adolescent girls with CSA. Using dance and movement therapy, I worked with the group as a psychosocial nurse over a period of ten weeks. The nursing interventions described herein were formulated as a result of my clinical experience with this group as well as theoretical and experiential knowledge I gained from an eight-month course, "The Use of Movement in Psychotherapy" (J. Castle, M. Hines, & P. Schick, personal communication, October 1991–May 1992).

The purpose of this chapter is to propose a creative nursing perspective to guide nurses in the therapeutic use of dance and movement with adolescents who have psychosocial difficulties resulting from a history of childhood sexual abuse (CSA).

CONCEPTUAL FRAMEWORK

The nursing intervention proposed here involves an intertwining of rational and creative processes. The nurse uses her intellectual capacity curing the assessment and intervention phases; however, in DMT, emphasis is on use of the creative process that dance and movement engages.

The theory of how creative process becomes engaged during therapy is drawn from Johnston's (1986) Model of Creative Causality; dance/movement is the particular creative modality being described for its psychotherapeutic value for clients with history of CSA. Childhood sexual abuse is viewed as a problem in a psychosocial context rather than acontextually as a clinical diagnosis. There is an expanded sense of what health is as an ongoing, dynamic, and creative process.

Johnston's vision of health, as defined in his Model of Creative Causality, centers around the concepts of aliveness and capacitance. Aliveness is the amount of creation present in a system (creation is anything brought into existence by the imagination, to cause to grow, to bring into being). Capacitance is the total amount of aliveness (life, vitality) a system is capable of embodying. In general, the CSA client is considered to have some diminishment of both aliveness and capacitance. The intervention proposed rests on the client's developing, through movement interaction with the nurse, some sense of the creative process, the creative possibility within herself. Through use of this creative process, the client ultimately will discover growth and healing.

Johnston's Model of Creative Causality

Johnston's model is built on three major concepts: (1) generative leaps, (2) enlivening, and (3) creative causality. Generative leaps is the idea that an organism reaches a point where it is unstable and no longer functioning well (such as the symptomatic client with CSA). At this point, the organism undergoes a transformative process—in this case, through the DMT nursing intervention—know as a generative leap, and emerges on the other side as a reorganized, fuller being with an increased capacity for continuing growth and change. In other words, after the dance/movement intervention, the CSA client has been transformed and now has a greater capacity for aliveness.

Enlivening, as defined by Johnston, is the multihued, evolutionary process of coming to full vibrancy. A metaphor would be to imagine a blank white piece of paper upon which gradually emerges one color, then another, then another, until a rainbow fills the page. When the nurse uses dance/movement to intervene with a client, she is actively engaging the process of enlivening in both herself and the client.

Creative causality is the idea that growth and development—in this case, of a human being—occur in an orderly, patterned fashion. However, the pattern evolves not linearly but dynamically; through the process of interplaying, unfolding patterns form. The symptoms that the CSA client experiences and manifests are viewed as having both a diminishing element (reducing the person's capacity for vitality and for moving toward form) and a protective element (shielding the person from that which she is not yet ready to handle). The DMT intervention is designed to facilitate the person's move through the growth stages toward a fuller, more formed sense of self.

Johnston's conceptualization of how the creative process unfolds in human beings follows two rhythms, the first half of which has four stages. The stages will be briefly outlined, along with a linkage to how a client with CSA might manifest each stage. It is important to note that humans can and do move back and forth among these stages, but it is believed that, at any given time, a person rests predominantly in one of them.

First Half of the Rhythm of Creation: Four Stages

Stage One: Precreation.   In this stage, the new impulse toward form lies incubating; this is the time before the appearance of creation in actual form. Reality in this stage is organized in the organismic, kinesthetic language of the body, the most elemental kind of knowing (Johnston, 1986, p. 18).

The symptomatic CSA client can and does at times revert to this stage. For example, the nurse might see a disintegration of the self where the "aliveness" of the person is very fragile and the biological level is close to the surface (the person sits curled on the floor, rocking gently, emanating a sense of animism). Psychologically, the client in this stage has difficulty handling major engagements with reality; the response instead is toward severe polarization or splitting. The creative process framework (Johnston, 1986; P. Schick, personal communication, March 1992) views such psychotic patterns as disintegration in the service of reclaiming the self. Here, the ability to make any boundary at all, such as the physical body's boundary between what's inside and outside, is in itself a boundary-making process. Thus, dissociation is viewed as the only way the person has to make a container for the self.

Stage Two: First Inspiration.   This stage is filled with "the magic and numinosity of the creative" (Johnston, 1986, p. 85). It is, again, the magic and wonder of early childhood and vivid imagination; the dominant language is a symbolic language of myth and metaphor. Playing, exploring, and pretending are vehicles for growth and discovery.

In the CSA client, the capacity to play, to imagine, to pretend are diminished. Research shows that the clearest differentiation of sexually abused from nonabused children comes when children are given five minutes of free play time: the abused child is quiet and placid and does not pretend and imagine (Lynch & Roberts, 1982).

In a DMT session with a CSA client during this stage, the client becomes aware, through the use of dance/movement, that there *is* an innate creative source in herself that she can access. The possibilities of "Aha! Maybe there *is* hope for me; maybe there is another way of being that I can discover!" come, palpably, into the room when clients are dancing together.

Stage Three: Stage of Struggle.   This stage leaves behind the magical and imaginative emphasis and engages in struggle; thus, feelings of loss can be strong here. The CSA client struggles against limits and toward establishing limits as a way of discovering who she is.

This stage is painfully manifested as the CSA client attempts to master a coherent sense of self. The ability to do so is repeatedly thwarted by recurrent nightmares, flashbacks, and overwhelming feelings of powerlessness (Finklehor, 1986). As the client begins to take on a sense of autonomy, she often confuses it with responsibility for the abuse itself. The overwhelming self-reproach that emerges is acted out aggressively either toward others or toward the self (Friedrich, 1990).

In the DMT intervention, this grappling stage is manifested when the client begins to realize the limitations of the therapist (e.g., the therapist is not always available) and of the therapy (e.g., there are still emotionally painful experiences to struggle with) and may result in behaviors such as coming late to class or refusing to move. Many of the movement metaphors may also reflect a theme of conflict.

Stage Four: Finished Forms.   In the last stage, the time of finishing and polishing, finished forms come into being. In the DMT therapeutic process, this is where major intrapersonal and interpersonal conflicts have been worked through and there is a sense of integrity and stability.

Second Half of the Rhythm: The Created Form in Context

Creative rhythm's second half involves interconnection of what has been created with the personal and social sources and contexts of that creation (Johnston, 1986, p. 90). For the CSA client engaged in dance/movement therapy, the intervention develops a more vital sense of self and enlarges her capacity to create flexible, dynamic, interpersonal relationships.

Johnston pointed out that human creative process "dances" among four languages—body, symbol, cognition, and emotions. Whereas most of Western medicine concentrates on the cognitive language, DMT joyfully incorporates all four ways of knowing. DMT begins with bodily knowing (that which is known through sensorimotor processes and experienced kinesthetically); it actively encourages use of images and metaphors; its theory base rests on the belief that the body in motion will call forth the language of the emotions. Finally, there is a time in DMT sessions for bringing to consciousness and into verbal form what was previously known only through movement, symbol, and emotion. The real art of DMT is to safely and gradually facilitate and integrate the dance among body, symbol, intellect, and emotion.

APPLICATION TO NURSING PRACTICE

Holistic Nursing: Creative, Embodied, and Rational

Expanding the nursing process to incorporate the psychotherapeutic use of dance/movement affords nursing the opportunity to interweave creative process theory, dance/movement therapy theory, and nursing theory. The creative nursing theory outlined here begins with Nightingale's (1860) premise that nursing concerns those activities that put the body in a position for healing to occur. What creative nursing adds is that the body is viewed as subject rather than object.

To that construct is added Peplau's (1952) theory that the essence of nursing is the relationship between nurse and client. Peplau's theory predominantly stresses the nurse's cognitive understanding of herself and her client; creative nursing adds that the nurse using dance/movement will bring her capacity for bodily knowing as well as intellectual knowing.

Creative nursing also draws from Watson's (1985) nursing theory, which posits that the nursing process goes beyond the physical body confined to time and space. To Watson's transpersonal caring construct, which states that the client's mind and emotions are routes to the inner self/soul, creative nursing adds that the person's body in motion is also a route to the inner self. It is posited here that the moving body of the client, in interaction with the bodily and cognitive knowing of the nurse-therapist, provides a powerful venue for integration of the physical, psychological, and emotional self.

As mentioned earlier, the particular population of concern in this chapter is adolescents with a history of CSA. The sexually abused person has an immediate need for physical and psychological safety. Via the DMT intervention, through the use of her body in movement, the person reshapes her personal experience around the body. In the process, there evolves a healing effect on the person's self-concept and capacity to relate healthily to others. Theory from three branches of DMT—(1) Chacian dance therapy, (2) authentic movement, and (3) creative/improvisational movement—will be woven throughout the description of the intervention.

Creative Nursing Intervention

The overall goal of the DMT intervention is to increase the person's capacity to experience the body as the source of creativity. The specific goals for the client with a history of CSA are directed toward changes in self-concept (physical self and personal self), affect regulation, and interpersonal relationships or interdependence.

Self-Concept. Generally, the nurse-therapist works first with the client's concept of the physical self. The therapist observes the client's body in motion and assesses the use and misuse of the body parts, breathing patterns, and tension. This information is then used to intervene with the individual in order to expand her ability to be more comfortable in her body and, later, to use the body more fully and appropriately for expression. The client seeks, slowly and progressively, to expand her capacity to simply experience the physical body and its senses. As she becomes increasingly able to experience her physical body in a positive way, her sense of body integrity expands and she can begin work on building a more realistic body image.

The client will concurrently be working on development of an autonomous, integrated sense of personal self. A central tenet of DMT theory is a belief that there is a constant, reciprocal interaction between body and mind (Schoop, 1974). More specifically, a change will come about in the person's self-concept as she expands her movement repertoire. To illustrate, after moving joyfully for several moments, one abused girl I worked with commented, "If I can feel this good moving, maybe there is hope for me after all."

One way in which the nurse-therapist using DMT can help the person shape or reshape her self-concept is to assist in experimentation with "effort qualities" of movement. The effort dimension of movement was articulated by Laban (1978), who described four motion factors—(1) flow, (2) weight, (3) time, and (4) space—that come together as a person moves.

The flow dimension involves the continuum between free, fluent ease of movement and bound/restrained flow in movement. The CSA client tends to be at one or the other extreme end of this continuum (either very rigid or completely boundless). The movement therapist assists her to develop flexibility: to use varying degrees of free or bound flow, depending on the situation, rather than to overuse one or the other.

The weight quality, ranging from light to strong, involves how the mover gets behind her weight and uses it to move. The CSA client often embodies strength as vehemence or as attack. Her embodying of lightness and gentleness often gets blurred with embodying compliance.

The time factor alternates between sustainment and suddenness; it is manifested in the way the mover shifts from one movement to another. The CSA client tends to evidence little quality of indulgence in time as she moves.

The space quality has to do with the mover's change in focus, either directly or indirectly, as she moves. The therapist is looking at a continuum in movement between a playfulness and a quality of concentration, or an ability to move playfully from one focus to another and then another. The CSA client tends to have limited capacity to find a balance between overconcentration and lack of any focus. To illustrate, one girl in my movement group said with sadness, "I can't just wander along, I just cannot do it, I start feeling lost, confused."

An understanding of these effort qualities has a real learning value for a client in terms of forming a healthy self-concept. She can ask herself: "Where in my life do I experience these qualities? Where are they absent or restricted in some way?" It is important for the nurse using movement/dance in therapy to make some assessment, together with the client, about where the person has access to these qualities and where there is room for growth and then for working with her on the latter.

Another way in which the dance therapist can work on development of personal self is to facilitate the mover's creating a personal movement metaphor (Levanthal & Chang, 1991). This process makes use of symbolic body action by encouraging the client to suggest images that evolve as she moves (Chaiklin & Schmais, 1979). The verbalization of the images encourages and crystallizes the movement. The nurse facilitates the connecting of the physical movement, mental image, and emotions by asking, for example: "What do you imagine in your life when you throw away what's no longer useful?"

Affect Regulation.   A basic theory of DMT is that dance/movement is the externalized form of inner feelings that cannot be rationally and verbally expressed. Further, it is believed that emotions form the bridge between the body and the psyche. Chodorow (1991) explained:

> *An emotion, by definition, is at once somatic and psychic. The somatic aspect is made up of bodily innervations and expressive physical action. The psychic aspect is made up of images and ideas. In psychopathology, the realms tend to split. By contrast, a naturally felt emotion involves a dialectical relationship—a union of body and psyche. (p. 3)*

A primary goal of dance/movement therapy is to facilitate the safe expression of affect. This is a particularly challenging goal when working with sexually abused clients, given their tendency for difficulty in affect regulation. The idea is to replace a client's fear and anger, frozen in her body and cut off from her self-knowledge, with a gradual experiencing of her body as powerful and in her control. As this process occurs through the dance/movement modality, the client learns to experience her feelings directly, own them, and express them appropriately rather than being overwhelmed by them.

It is a given of dance/movement therapy that affect may sponta-neously erupt out of a movement process. The first step in ensur-ing that this happens safely is to establish trust between therapist and client. With the CSA client, the nurse-therapist's role is not to rescue her but to provide emotional support and to offer valida-tions of her experience. As the mover's story unfolds, the therapist offers support by gradually providing here-and-now reinforcement when necessary. ("You are here with [therapist's name], you are safe, feel the support of the floor beneath your feet.") The thera-pist may also physically provide boundaries by, for example, plac-ing her back against the mover's back.

The therapist may also invite support from other group members and verbalize to the mover what others are doing to support her. (In a group that has been working together for a while, this will occur spontaneously.) Then the therapist provides quiet time for integration. The group may choose to do some journaling or draw-ing prior to a verbal discussion of the movement session.

Well-handled, the expression of intense affect can be very heal-ing for the client. I am reminded of an occasion when a client in my movement group began to experience intense anger during her moving. With support from the group, she continued to move; gradually, her movements became those of a person taking control of her body rather than being controlled. Following the move-ment, the girl drew a vivid picture of a red and black spider; she explained that this represented her abuser. She then stood up and stomped directly on the spider. Later, she told me that, in her ver-bal psychotherapy groups, she was able to directly articulate her anger and connect it with her abuser rather than taking it inward against herself.

Interdependence.   Through the DMT container, wherein development of trust is primary, the client is actively working on her capacity for mutually reinforcing interpersonal relationships. As with any psychotherapy, the therapist begins with promoting trust. Marian Chace led the DMT field in the task of how to develop a therapeutic relationship on a movement level. She mastered the art of mirroring, which involves an understanding (on both visual and kinesthetic levels) of what the client is expressing in movement terms. Through the movement of her body, Chace would expand, reflect back, or make more complete a client's tentative movement (Chaiklin & Schmais, 1979). Through this movement process, the therapist communicates acceptance and understanding. Thus, empathy in movement terms is established and a foundation of trust is built.

When working on interpersonal issues, the Chacian group format works toward the goals of reinforcing unity and decreasing alienation and loneliness. The nurse-therapist facilitates the development of group movement metaphors in order to bring out and work through interpersonal issues. As outlined by Levanthal and Chang (1991), the therapist directs movers: "Find a movement that feels alive and right for you at this time." As clients begin moving, she reminds them: "Retain the central core of your own movement." After several minutes, she remarks: "One-by-one, you will form a whole. You have the option to make physical contact or not." She guides movers: "Pay attention to what shifts in you and how it occurs when you change your movement to accommodate the whole group." Ideally, the movers discover their own movement metaphors, and the theme emerges from the client group.

The therapist must choose her words, images, and movement directives carefully, allowing room for individual expression (Levanthal & Chang, 1991). For example, there is a big difference in what happens when the therapist says, "Punch the creep!" and what happens when she says, "Use your arms and legs noisily and use all your weight and all the space in the room." It is a complex goal—and the real art of the dance/movement therapist—to encourage group cohesion and feelings of belonging all the while supporting the maintenance of a personal sense of identity.

Role of the Nurse Using Dance/Movement

The nurse-therapist described in this chapter should have a Master's degree and special training in the use of movement in psychotherapy. Her role is to facilitate innate creative process, as described above. She directs the mover to a fuller, more embodied self where her physical, imaginal, emotional, and cognitive realms are increasingly more integrated. To facilitate in a safe and supportive way, the nurse must herself have a "center of being," that is, an integrated sense of self. Only with a secure sense of self can the nurse using dance/movement provide the necessary container within which the mover can feel safe. In addition to the interpersonal, metaphysical container, the nurse provides structure through selecting a specific time, place, and consistent therapist for the sessions.

The nurse-therapist also has an important role in delivering ongoing feedback to the mover regarding intrapersonal and interpersonal movement characteristics. Regarding individual feedback about physical movement, the nurse attempts to focus on her own response to a particular movement so that the client is free to own the feedback or not. For example, "When you did this [describe movement], this moved in me [describe]"; or "When you bent your head to your chest and curled your arms around your center, a very young place in me was moved." This response offers a "witnessing" of the mover without judgment and heightens the recognition of the process as a transpersonal one. The nurse will more fully facilitate the process if she allows time for quiet, natural integration following each movement experience.

Structure of Group Sessions

In my movement therapy group of adolescent girls, the following structure worked well for a 45-minute session. We began with a 5-minute warm-up session in which we did gentle stretching and rhythmic movement around peripheral body parts, such as wiggling the toes, massaging the feet, patting the knees, clapping the hands. We then moved into a circle and began actively moving together. I would lead a movement and then individual group members would lead in the Chacian "pass the movement" tradition. Next came active group movement during which a group theme emerged and was expanded. This was followed by a slower, cooldown closure segment, generally ending with stretching and relaxation. Depending on what had transpired in the session, we would have a verbal discussion or quiet time to put the experience into more concrete form (i.e., journaling, clay modeling, drawing) prior to discussion.

CONCLUSION

Dance/movement therapy, which honors interconnections among the body, the mind, and the emotions, offers a valuable means of interweaving the cognitive and the embodied creative process into nursing theory, research, and practice. Using DMT as a nursing intervention is particularly appropriate with clients who have psychosocial difficulties following the experience of CSA.

The implications for nursing practice, however, go beyond one particular clinical population. DMT has the potential to have positive impact on many populations that are of concern to nursing, such as those with affective disorders and those with developmental disorders. Because it is based on an overall model of creative process, DMT is particularly appropriate for nursing interventions with children and adolescents.

The use of DMT as a nursing intervention has rarely been the subject of nursing research. An example of the recommended research is to test the impact of the use of DMT on the self-esteem, body image, and relationship patterns of adolescent girls with a history of CSA.

To that first group of clients I saw moving, back on Fifth Hall; to the adolescent girls described in this chapter, with whom it has been my privilege to work; and to those with whom I shall work in the future, I say: Let the dance continue!

REFERENCES

Chaiklin, S., & Schmais, C. (1979). The Chace approach to dance therapy. In P. L. Bernstein (Ed.), *Eight theoretical approaches to dance/ movement therapy* (pp. 15–30). Dubuque, IA: Kendall/Hunt.

Chodorow, J. (1991). *Dance therapy and depth psychology.* New York: Routledge & Kegan Paul.

Finklehor, D. (1986). *A sourcebook on child sexual abuse.* Beverly Hills, CA: Sage.

Friedrich, W. N. (1990). Psychotherapy of sexually abused children and their families. New York: W. W. Norton.

Johnston, C. M. (1986). *The creative imperative.* Berkeley, CA: Celestial Arts.

Kestenberg, J., & Sossin, M. (1979). *The role of movement patterns in development II.* New York: Dance Notation Bureau.

Laban, R. (1978). *Modern educational dance.* London: MacDonald & Evans.

Levanthal, F., & Chang, M. (1991). Dance/movement therapy with battered women: A paradigm of action. *American Journal of Dance Therapy, 13*(2), 131–145.

Lynch, M. A., & Roberts, J. (1982). *Consequences of child abuse.* New York: Academic Press.

Nightingale, F. (1860). *Notes on nursing: What it is and what it is not.* London: Harrison & Sons.

Peplau, H. (1952). *Interpersonal relations in nursing.* New York: Putnam.

Roy, C. (1976). *Introduction to nursing: An adaptation model.* Englewood Cliffs, NJ: Prentice-Hall.

Schmais, C. (1974). Dance therapy in perspective. In K. C. Mason (Ed.), *Dance Therapy* (Focus on Dance, VII). Washington, D.C.: American Association of Health, Education and Recreation.

Schoop, T. (1974). *Won't you join the dance?* Palo Alto, CA: National Press Books.

Watson, J. (1985). *Nursing: Human science and human care.* Norwalk, CT: Appleton-Century-Crofts.

Part IV

Art as Reflective Experience

16

Kate Millett's Loony-Bin Trip: Reflections and Implications for Nursing

Wanda K. Mohr

A number of years ago, Kate Millett, the radical feminist scholar, author, and artist, published the story of her struggle to maintain her humanity in the enslaving and toxic environment of contemporary psychiatric "care." That passionate and linguistically exquisite tale, *The Loony-Bin Trip,* is so profound a work that further description is very much in danger of being shallow or superficial. Readers of this chapter should perhaps go on to experience the story directly.

Excerpts from *The Loony-Bin Trip* reprinted by permission of Simon & Schuster, New York. Copyright © 1990 by Kate Millett.

This chapter is dedicated to Beverly H. Hall, PhD, RN, who always cared and inspired.

Yet to relegate this valuable narrative to the realm of private experience is to deny the oppressed group whom we label as "mentally ill" an eloquent and publicly articulated exemplar of what it means to be mentally ill in society today. Those who have been so labeled can take heart from Millett's affirmation. Nurses who want to work with the mentally ill would do well to understand, from their clients' point of view, the kind of devastation that good intentions and distorted "caring" can produce.

This chapter presents an interpretation of six passages from Millett's story by applying some principles from Norman Denzin's (1989) interpretive interactional approach to qualitative analysis. In presenting this analysis, the author hopes to illustrate how works of art can be used as heuristic methods in teaching and in exploring the meaning of a patient's condition. The passages that have been chosen for interpretation are representative of Millett's existential text and exemplify her experience on her journey and her struggle for personal transcendence.

ANALYTIC APPROACH

In analyzing a narrative as rich as *The Loony-Bin Trip,* an interpretive approach such as that advocated by Denzin (1989) is particularly salient. Denzin asserted that the interpretive approach should be used when a researcher wishes to examine relationships between personal troubles and the public policies and institutions that have been created to address those personal troubles. He suggested that, all too frequently, social programs are formulated by well-meaning individuals (experts) based on faulty or incorrect understanding of the human condition of those whom they purport to serve. The horror experienced by Millett stands as testament to Denzin's contention that many programs do not work precisely because they are constructed on a failure to take into account the perspective and attitude of the person served. Millett's story is an intensely damning indictment of a mental health system that confines those whom society has cast out as "mad."

Central among the features of Denzin's method is the contextualized interpretation of thick descriptions—those that convey meaning and experiences in a richly detailed manner as opposed to a simple recording of facts. The process of contextualization in the interpretation of these descriptions is based on Mills's (1959) notion of the sociological imagination. Mills's idea is that such imagination will enable the scholar to grasp history and biography and the relation between the two.

An additional feature of interpretive interaction is its emphasis on the epiphany—an experience in a person's life that leaves a profound mark and has the potential for transformation of that life (Denzin, 1989). Millett's experience with the mental health system was most certainly an epiphany for her. A study of her experiences comes very close to being an epiphany of sorts for her readers as well.

THE STORY

The setting is Millett's art colony for women, which she has founded on a farm in Poughkeepsie, New York. She has decided to stop lithium, which she has been taking for a number of years. The decision was made in collaboration with her lover, Sophie, and was made known to the other women at the colony. She begins writing in a quasi-stream-of-consciousness (Millett, 1990):

For they love us, as we love them, every day more so, friendship becoming a drunkedness becoming love, a love none of us define, so we call it the farm or the colony, as if it were merely an idea, an ideology of a communal something politically correct. Through it, rapturously happy . . .

Life has never been so good. The apprentices, the farm, the summer still only ahead, only half over, spreading already to a richness, a perfection, like a peony in full bloom. Or the loosestrife around the pond. And Sophie. All, I have everything. I am even off the lithium. With no ill effects. It is six weeks now and we have been keeping check on the experiment, and if it works I am whole. Either I was never crazy or I have recovered and can be sane henceforth. To be whole, not a cracked egg, not an imperfect specimen, not

a deformed intellect or a mental defective—but whole.
(pp. 16-17)

In this passage, Millett suggests a possibility of authenticity and human connectedness that defies words. In her love of Sophie, which extends exponentially to "the others," she has a glimmer of the pristine—the hallowing of the commonplace (farm), the unaffected blending of the ecstatic and the quotidian, the fostering of genuine community. The passage shimmers with love, not only in the context of her feelings for Sophie and "the others," but also in tentative relation to herself. She has stopped taking a medication that has marked her as a blemished "specimen."

At the same time, there are hints of foreshadowing of problems ahead in the mention of the "loosestrife." Although loosestrife is a tree, the deliberate mention of it in this passage seems to suggest the conflicts to come. An additional portent may be insinuated in the image of the cracked egg, which brings to mind the idea of Humpty Dumpty and his fall from a wall.

After an episode of anger during which she becomes frustrated with her insurance company and lashes out at the apprentices over a minor transgression, Millett phones her sister, an attorney, to discuss her difficulties. Her sister's response is to ask her whether she is taking her lithium. Millett (1990) writes:

> *Suddenly it all comes back, the last time, the loony-bin trip, the shame, the terror of being locked up. It was she who put me there—a thing I can forgive, but not quite forget, thought it was forgotten until the lime: "Are you taking your medicine?" Like a bullying sergeant, like an order, like a prison guard in those prisons I thought I had left forever. I realize that if she were to know I have gone off the stuff, she might be out here in no time, might even have me busted with a few phone calls. Meaning well—they always mean well. And they always win . . . (p. 28)*

This passage is replete with the intensity of Millett's remembered fear of being a prisoner, of having her will subjugated to her sister, who assumes an oppressing military posture with her question-accusation. Millett recalls being ashamed at having her freedom taken away. Being judged by others to be too incompetent to remain within society must have been profoundly humiliating to a scholar of Millett's stature. There is also a suggestion that it is a shameful thing to attribute nefarious motives to a loved one who only "means well."

Gradually, Millett (1990) comes to the realization that "the others" are beginning to doubt her sanity and her life seems to be an endless disputation with Sophie about whether she should or should not start taking her lithium again:

> And now the joy had disappeared altogether in arguments and quarrels between Sophie and me. At the end of it I feel my back against the wall and the circle forming around me, the accusations of madness. That I am not quite right, that something has come over me in the last two weeks, some terrible change. "People would hardly know you," the solemn approach. "You're a little freaked out," the hip diagnosis. And the ones behind my back whispering that this is an attack she's having, she's flipped out. How little weight my own perceptions seem to have. I am the discussed . . . (p. 72)

The final sentence in this section suggests the profound alienation that Millett has begun to experience. She has ceased to be a person, and has become the object of the scrutiny of "the others." They have found the fights draining, and, like lemmings, have schooled together. She feels isolated and trapped. Her relations with others have become impersonal, detached, superficial, limited only to either direct or covert allusions to her state of mind. They have lost any connection to her as a person of individual identity beneath the abstract schematization of the quasi-diagnostic labels our society uses to partition those who are unfortunate enough to be mentally ill.

Millett (1990) makes an attempt to reestablish the bond that she had with Sophie:

I had asked her to caress me, to make love to me a few moments so I could sleep, so the terror would go away, so the fury would stay put, so that my spine could unclench it-self—because I so desperately needed to sleep. I begged her and she would not, was not in the mood and couldn't put herself there. "Only so that I can sleep, please touch me." "No." (p. 83)

Millett's isolation becomes complete with Sophie's final rejection. The word "begged" suggests the magnitude of her need for human contact. In the end, the Oxford scholar is reduced to entreating her friend for a single touch to allay her fear and panic, to soothe her dread and allow her to sleep. She is rejected.

Millett's well-meaning friends and family attempt to have her committed when she returns to New York City at summer's end, but fail when she invokes her civil rights. However, on a trip to Ireland in support of political prisoners, she is picked up at the airport in Dublin at the request of her family and "friends." Her passport is confiscated and she is interned in a public psychiatric institution where she is forcibly given lithium and Thorazine. She is denied visitors and any contact with the outside world. When she attempts to escape and the staff discovers that she is cheeking her medications, Prolixin is added to her medication regime. Her life begins to resemble a phantasmorphic, nightmarish daze.

In her narration of her incarceration in this hospital, no one escapes Millett's relentlessly frank description of the horror of her stay. The physicians are authoritarian, condescending, and lacking in any warmth, compassion, or even human respect. No less deficient are the staff nurses, who are portrayed as obtuse and robotic.

In a particularly poignant description of a group therapy activity, Millett recounts how journaling and letter writing are promoted as a therapeutic activity intended for catharsis and self expression. She later discovers that these results of patients' labors are being destroyed and never read by the staff in the interest of "patient confidentiality." This metaphor of a client's hopes, dreams, and healthy impulses being summarily nullified by a toxic and indifferent bureaucracy is devastating in its implications.

Nevertheless, her indomitable spirit prevails, always calling on her creativity and knowledge of her own integrity, and she never yields to the system. Her politically active Irish friends finally track her down and she is released from this horror with the help of an iconoclastic psychiatrist.

Upon returning to New York City, Millett (1990) experiences a profound depression:

> *Depression is death . . . (p. 257)*
>
> *During depression the world disappears. Language itself. One has nothing to say. Nothing. No small talk, no anecdotes . . . The loss of language is so crucial, such a bereavement. Language does not really go away, it goes inward. Downward. Shriveling in the process, becoming repetitious, as when one facing great peril repeats that same protective formulas. Yet one mourns language, sociability, camaraderie, needing it now more than ever. And how necessary it becomes just as one observes its superficiality, the wavering of friends, the coldness of strangers, the essential uncaring of life itself, its monstrosity. And in the face of this evil—not even to have words to protect one from the volume. To grow mute as well as helpless. (pp. 283-284)*

The phenomenon of being without words must be understood in the context of Millett's being a writer and a professor of literature and philosophy, on the one hand, and simply a person on the other. She has lost the power of words, and words are her means of livelihood; they are also the means by which she has made her mark on the literary world and the instrument for her passionate struggle for the liberation of people.

As a person, she has lost connection with community and with others through the loss of her ability to communicate. Even the possibility of pseudo-community, which supposedly includes everyone but offers a living encounter with no one, has vanished with the appearance of "the theme of silence." Millett has become mute in the face of the overwhelming force of a limit situation. In her depression, she likens the experience to death.

She seeks help from a private psychiatrist whom she has consulted in the past, but is unable to tolerate his smug and patronizing attitude. She is rapidly becoming financially impoverished. At this point in her story, a profound epiphany occurs.

In desperation, she goes to a "charity" hospital's emergency room where she becomes one of the "sick and destitute." Here, among the "shabby," she begins to attain an elementary communion with another person, Benfield, a bland and good-natured psychiatric resident. Benfield, in his uncomplicated honesty and nonjudgmental acceptance, soothes her. In addition, her presence among "this alienated sea of humanity" in the emergency room brings an elemental and sober authenticity into her life.

In a hauntingly indeterminate way, she begins to recover:

> *But the blossoms on the trees, the heat of the sidewalk, the insistence of spring in the warmth of the stucco, the push of the new leaves . . . I am getting better. (p. 314)*

The remainder of Millett's book deals with her decision to stop taking lithium and essentially regain control over the integrity of her mind and over her life. In writing about her experiences, she affirms the inviolability of the human mind and pleads for tolerance for mental activity at the margin. Her work rejects the notion that the ever-expanding mastery of facts and the objectification of humans will eventually lead to an optimal state of well-being or adjustment.

CONCLUDING THOUGHTS

The year 1992 brought a number of inquiries by legislative and state regulatory agencies into the practices of private psychiatric hospitals and their treatment of patients. Testimony by former patients, families, and "medical" experts ranged from allegations of kidnapping and people being held against their will, to unnecessary admissions (Staff, Texas State Senate Interim Committee, 1992). It would seem reasonable that nurses, as employees of these hospitals, would have known of these practices; yet the Board of

Nurse Examiners in Texas reported that virtually no reports of these practices had been received (Staff, 1992).

The nursing profession clearly delineates safeguarding the client as a key element in its code of ethics (1985). Yet, just as clearly, nurses failed to live up to their mandate to act as advocates of their clients. The reasons for this failure may be rooted in the patriarchal and hierarchical nature of our oppressive "medical" institutions. Even so, one is led to confront the question: "What happened to our humanity?" In the 1940s, 1960s, and 1970s, essays and books appeared that documented the continued debasing conditions in "mental" hospitals (Deutch, 1948; Goffman, 1961; Rosenhan, 1973). Based on the nursing research done by Morrison (1990), which documents a "tradition of toughness" as a norm on a psychiatric unit, conditions for clients have changed very little over the decades.

It would behoove us as a profession to take a very long, measured, and critical look at what has happened in nursing with respect to the psychiatric hospital scandal. We are obliged to our profession, to ourselves, and most especially to our clients to try to find answers as to why nurses remained silent in the face of what was so obviously patient abuse. More importantly, we must ensure that such things never happen again for they seriously diminish us as a profession and as people.

We must begin at an elementary level to speculate as to the reasons behind nursing's behavior, even as we conduct research studies to determine what nurses were experiencing in these environments. Perhaps they did not have the tools with which to advocate for their clients and for their profession. Perhaps nursing education has so completely bought into the dominant empiricist paradigm of the medical model that it has effectively educated us as technicians, but just as effectively has robbed us of our capacity for creative, critical thinking, ethical decision making, and autonomy.

For a number of years, nursing scholars have called for a revolution in the way nurses are taught (Bevis & Murray, 1990; Donley, 1989; Moccia, 1989). This visionary call to a curriculum that would include a greater exploration of qualitative methods such as phenomenology, hermeneutical analysis, and poetics preceded the scandals in the psychiatric hospitals by a number of years. What these scholars were seeking to avoid in terms of "creeping dehumanization" may have been realized, as the scandal has dramatically illustrated.

If we can see this as an opportunity for self-appraisal, we must also see that it can portend a new and important time in our nursing history and nursing education, a time when we can move beyond a concern with occupational clutter and prescribed patterns of behavior. We must begin to refocus our vision on humanity and seek new ways of gaining insight into the human condition. One way might be by revolutionizing nursing curricula to include the humanities, literature, history, and art as tools for exploring the ontological connections among all people. Great literature can be a self-evident source of instruction, for it informs the mind and heart through an emotional engagement with characters who can beautifully articulate their most personal experiences.

Analyses and readings like *The Loony-Bin Trip* can provide valuable material for the understanding of a client's experience of mental illness that no psychopharmacology, psychobiology or DSM-III-R-based course in psychiatric nursing can ever begin to approach.

We owe our clients nothing less than the deepest understanding of them and of their experiences that we can achieve.

REFERENCES

American Nurses Association. (1985). *Code book for nurses with interpretive statements.* Kansas City, MO: Author.

Bevis, E. O., & Murray, J. P. (1990). The essence of the curriculum revolution: Emancipatory teaching. *Journal of Nursing Education, 29,* 326–331.

Denzin, N. (1989). *Interpretive interactionism.* Newbury Park, CA: Sage.

Deutch, A. (1948). *The shame of the states.* New York: Harcourt, Brace.

Donley, S. R. (1989). Curriculum revolution: Heeding the voices of change. In *Curriculum revolution: Reconceptualizing nursing education* (pp. 1–8). New York: National League for Nursing.

Goffman, E. (1961). *Asylums: Essays on the social situation of mental patients and other inmates.* Garden City, NY: Doubleday.

Millett, K. (1990). *The loony-bin trip.* New York: Simon & Schuster.

Mills, C. W. (1959). *The sociological imagination.* New York: Oxford University Press.

Moccia, P. (1989). Curriculum reconceptualization: Integrating the voices of revolution. In *Reconceptualizing nursing education* (pp. 135-144). New York: National League for Nursing.

Morrison, E. F. (1990). The tradition of toughness: A study of nonprofessional nursing care in psychiatric settings. *Image: The Journal of Nursing Scholarship, 22*(1), 32-38.

Rosenhan, D. L. (1973, January). On being sane in insane places. *Science, 179,* 250-257.

Staff, (1992, February). Senate interim committee studies private psychiatric and substance abuse services. *R.N. Update,* 1.

Staff, Texas State Senate Interim Committee. (1992, November). *Report on private psychiatric, substance abuse, and medical rehabilitation services.* Austin, TX.

Night Shift in the ICU
Wanda K. Mohr

Nursing, I think, is an ethereal whisper
Of joining . . . of two
Gentle as the shimmer of early morning dew
Strong as a steadying touch
Amid the cacophonous screech of daily chaos

Sometimes after midnight or in the muted early hours
I sit dutifully assembling requisite dispassionate words
They appear, disembodied, in the neat slant of Palmer.
I ponder their form and marvel at the lack of content
While I gather the solitude of the night
Like a cloak
And fiercely listen beyond the machines

The voice an image of sound, anguish, loneliness,
  fear . . . here
"Nurse . . . please."

Then silence, motionless sound
A look
Seismic eyes darting
Like the frantic oscillations on the screen of the heart,
Hoary, ragged breathing each carefully engrafted
With its own numerical indicator.

Beyond the arachnoid prison of lines that precisely drop
  nutrition,
Comes a wisdom that guides.
I begin, "What . . . ?"
Approximate words.
The answer comes . . . "No, just be . . . with me"
And we are
Changed for all time in that moment.

17

Aesthetics and Memories: Pathway to Synthesis of a Dialectic

Mary Hobbs Leenerts

*I*n the evening of the day, a woman is crossing a narrow bridge alone. The fog is settling in around her, and the mist is cool on her face. She looks out on the darkening horizon, and memories engage her. She connects with images of the past, searching for relationships that will strengthen her and offer hope for facing doubt and uncertainty. Both have become her constant companions, a part of her being. This flood of memories represents a kind of ontological work, a kind of ontological imaging, in which she connects with mental images that hint of her own transforming. Recently, her memories have connected with images that strengthen her for facing her own death. She is struggling to find meaning in life while facing death, a death that will most certainly come, because she is living with AIDS.

Dying has been described as a developmental phenomenon of evolving consciousness representing a transformation of the person's energy pattern (Schorr, 1983). In this process, the dying person may or may not develop a participatory relationship with death. The woman who is walking alone and is living in the questioning is participating in a relationship with death. She is intimately involved in the dialectic relationship of living while dying. In her imagery, she encounters "unclear shadows." She struggles to discover the personal meaning of this experience and to practice her own ways of "letting go" of the old and coconstructing the new. She images ways of being in this life experience. This ontological imaging guides her as she faces existential issues and participates in the coconstruction of meaning while living in the paradox between life and death.

Sarter (1987) discussed evolutionary idealism and the view that human conscious energy evolves to ever higher complexity. This is compatible with Schorr's (1983) suggestion that evolving consciousness represents a transformation of energy; the human being is not the final stage in this evolving consciousness. As the woman images her reality and attempts to cocreate meaning in her experience, she finds herself asking questions that revolve around the discovery of self-reality.

As she searches for her self-reality, she is struggling to answer the question: "Who am I now that I am living with this disease process?" This reflexive questioning guides her in restructuring her world-view and in choosing what is valued. She chooses and acts on values, seeking meaning all-at-once. She is living the paradoxical unity of revealing–concealing (self), enabling–limiting (choices for self-care), and connecting–separating (within relationships). These rhythmical patterns of engagement, described by Parse (1981), provide the ontological dimension for living in life's paradoxes.

As the woman engages in reflexivity around self and meaning, she experiences a dialectic of movement between inner and outer experience. Zaner (1981) focused on reflexivity and wonder in self-development and suggested that, inwardly, the self shows itself as a situated reflexivity within its own embodied subjective life. It has two foundational moments: "its own whereby it is itself and alone, and its urgency to let itself be manifested outwardly, to 'ek-sist' in the environing milieu for and along with other selves" (Zaner, 1981, p. 152). Zaner described the self as present to itself from the beginning but not already awakened to itself. This happening of self-awakening or self-recognition is an unfolding of what was always and already present and is characterized by encounter, disclosure, emergence, and discovery. In Zaner's view, the self's reflexivity operates in the dialectic between inner and outer experience.

The woman's esthetic ontological experience is cued into: (1) what has happened to her life-world, (2) what she is experiencing, (3) what skills are required, and (4) the possibilities for action (Benner & Wrubel, 1989). As the woman faces these ontological cues, essences can be extracted from her story. She is close to images of vulnerability and loss as she expresses grief over a missed future. Around death are images requiring emotional energy for facing a bridge that looms over the future. She is aware that she is walking new lifeways as certainty and uncertainty blend to reveal a changing self. She feels frozen and changing all-at-once while forcing herself to engage in self-care practices.

Within this self-reflexivity, the woman is focused on engaging possibilities for originating patterns that free her to change in the transforming. Finding time to play with mental images and the feelings these images evoke allows for a rehearsal of possibilities and for empowerment through imagery. This imagery work is consistent with ways of finding meaning within ontological phenomenology as described by Heidegger (1968). Imaginative rehearsal represents an application of Heideggerian ontological phenomenology. It is characterized by facing what lies before one—listening to tacit and cognitive knowing and allowing both ways of knowing to lead the way of being. It is a participation in the metaphysical dimension of being. It is a responding to the "call," the "invitation" into a relationship, a presence with one's own being (Heidegger, 1968). We are "invited" into a relationship, a presence with our very own nature. Visualization or imagery influences mental consciousness (Sarter, 1987) and provides a pathway for engaging in a relationship of presence with our very own nature.

Because of time's influence, the process of coconstituting meaning is ongoing. For the woman, feelings of self-change were linked with a spiritual connection. Imagery helped her to move toward practices of peace, prayer, love, and relationship within community. She described practicing peace and love techniques until one day these practices seemed to be automatic and there was a change in feeling. Sarter (1987) suggested that meditation and prayer influence spiritual consciousness and that spiritual consciousness permeates all levels of conscious energy. Reed (1992) described spirituality as connectedness that is integral to human development. This interconnectedness has intrapersonal, interpersonal, and transpersonal dimensions. Spiritual care is described as part of the ontologic foundation of nursing (Reed, 1992). Spirituality is a pathway for transformation beyond the physical. Nursing's emerging paradigm on spirituality is a pattern of wholeness and connectedness (Reed, 1992).

From listening to this woman's story, patterns emerged that have implications for holistic nursing care. In the first pattern, individual stories are recognized and valued, and they become central to coparticipating with memory work and imagery that empowers. This valuing of life stories and coparticipating in memory work can be empowering to patient, nurse, and significant others. Active play with the person's imaging mobilizes creative energy.

The second pattern is a pattern of rehearsal of ways of preferred being. When this rehearsal includes self-care and choices about enabling self-care, an empowering experience may follow. Rehearsal on the imaginary ontologic stage helps prepare for possibilities in the ontologic reality. By helping persons identify self-care practices, both physical and emotional, self-care can be empowered. The purpose of this originating of ways of being is to enable healthy self-care in a variety of life experiences.

The third pattern involves living through uncertainty and chaos with the trust that order will evolve. There is recognition that changing or transforming is a part of the evolution of consciousness. The focus is on helping the person connect with change through living with the ambiguity of change. One way to do this might be through the use of life story with emphasis on how changing manifests, and how one might connect with meaning and creativity in that process. Engagement in caring relationships and coparticipation in making and perpetuating shared memories are central to supporting spirituality and holistic patterns of nursing care.

Deikman (1971) has described action and receptive modes of consciousness as a bimodal pattern of consciousness. The action mode involves goal-directed behavior and is futurist and individual in orientation. The receptive mode is oriented to inner openness, to intake of the environment, and to the present. Schorr (1983) suggested that persons who rely on the action mode may or may not be aware that they are more than a corporeal entity. In Western culture, ritual and rites of passage do not guide the death experience, and there is little understanding of human energy patterns and evolving consciousness within persons facing death. The woman walking on the bridge has within her the resources to determine her own ritual and rite of passage through the death experience. In her reflexive inquiry, she is engaging the receptive mode of consciousness and is participating in the enhancement of her evolution of consciousness.

In the intrapersonal dynamics of the human health experience of death, nurses can help facilitate the action and receptive modes of consciousness. In this supportive connection, the action and receptive modes of the life–death dialectic can be synthesized into a holistic state of evolving consciousness. Weaving a story within the memories is one way the woman attempts to live with certainty–uncertainty within living–dying. In weaving her story, she manifests the bimodal pattern of consciousness while moving between action in the outer life-world and receptive openness in the inner life-world.

Boykin and Schoenhofer (1991) suggested that story is the link among nursing practice, ontology, and epistemology. This supports the perspective that self-narratives are necessary to recognize/understand patterns that reveal the relational self and the evolution of consciousness. Story provides an esthetic method for organizing and communicating nursing knowledge about this woman's experience of living the life–death dialectic.

As the woman reaches the end of the bridge, her story reflects moments of memories encompassing a lifetime. The story expresses her concerns about making her way through the experience of living–dying. She images this experience and reaches for words to articulate its meaning:

> *When I'm dying, please don't speak to me of closure. Don't speak to me of things undone and making final plans, and doing end things. I haven't thought of closure as I've faced my life . . . and death. To me, the useful concept is connection. Speak to me of connecting in ways that touch the spiritual . . . that blend memories with the ethereal in the inner workings that know forever. When I'm dying, please don't speak to me of closure . . . allow me to connect with what is forever . . . memories that transcend the going.*

In nursing care, if we lose sight of being and focus on epistemology to the expense of ontology, we may block ontological images and memory work. It is possible that we interfere with the spiritual connection and patterns of spirituality. Ontology can be captured in the relationship; epistemology grows through expanded understanding of the meaning of relationship. Relationships are important because they reveal connectedness, context, and time, all characteristics of pattern (Newman, 1986).

Processes in the evolution of consciousness and in ontological imaging and memory work are bound to aesthetics. The nurse who values holistic practices will coparticipate with persons on the pathway of living life while facing death. The nurse will support the person's unique ways of synthesizing this dialectic by helping connect with the story through memories and images that support the transformation of evolving consciousness.

EPILOGUE

In the aesthetic experience of weaving images and memories into story, the nurse supports the patient's evolutionary process of consciousness. The following poem represents an attempt to capture the importance of coparticipating with persons in their evolution of consciousness in the dialectic of living with death.

Memories

Memories like shadows come and go.
   And in the going . . .
   what happens to this lifetime?
When there is no more form.
   And the pattern is gone . . .
   or seems to be gone.
Maybe memories like shadows play.
   And run and jump in illusive games . . .
   in a theater of their own.
Still claiming ethereal privileges.
   On a stage beyond . . .
   where memories and shadows have gone.
Watching those within this lifetime.
   Reach to palpate their soul . . .
   to touch memories within the shadow show.

REFERENCES

Benner, P., & Wrubel, J. (1989). *The primacy of caring.* Menlo Park, CA: Addison-Wesley.

Boykin, A., & Schoenhofer, S. O. (1991). Story as link between nursing practice, ontology, epistemology. *Image: The Journal of Nursing Scholarship, 23*(4), 245-248.

Deikman, J. J. (1971). Bimodal consciousness. *Archives of General Psychiatry, 25,* 418-489.

Heidegger, M. (1968). *What is called thinking? (Was Heisst Denken?,* J. G. Gray, Trans.). New York: Harper & Row.

Newman, B. (1986). *Health as expanding consciousness.* St. Louis: Mosby.

Parse, R. R. (1981). *Man-living-health: A theory of nursing.* New York: Wiley.

Reed, P. G. (1992). An emerging paradigm for the investigation of spirituality in nursing. *Research in Nursing and Health, 15,* 349-357.

Sarter, B. (1987). Evolutionary idealism: A philosophical foundation for holistic nursing theory. *Advances in Nursing Science, 9*(2), 1-9.

Schorr, J. A. (1983). Manifestations of consciousness and the developmental phenomenon of death. *Advances in Nursing Science, 6*(1), 26–35.

Zaner, R. M. (1981). *The context of self.* Athens: Ohio University Press.

To The Wounded Healer: A Nurse Researcher Responds
Joanne Marky Supples

I have seen your face
A hundred faces in a thousand shadows
The face of sadness from the dim past
That emerges as the pain is felt again
And again, the remedy invites relief
From the memory of old atrocities

I have heard your story
A hundred stories in a thousand voices
Crying out in silence and in pain
From injuries some known some buried deep
That come to surface pain again, again
And calls you back to the old remedy

I have felt your pain
A pain so exquisite I dare not touch
A pain received for no warranted cause
As infant, child, virginal youth
And with you I cry out for all to hear
What remedy replaces human love?

I have seen your pain
In dear innocent faces
In loss of hope and fear to try
In cut up skin and bleeding hearts
In tortured bodies large and small,
Women and men in white atoning
For sins of others not their own.
What remedy replaces human care?

I know your pain and know your loss, I care.
Beyond the common way of caring, intimately knowing
No sin, no fault of yours, no crime but ours
Forgive our blind deceit and harsh retort
You are the hero who survives
A holocaust of yet unknown toll and
Guilty bystanders.

Take heart, dear colleague,
Not victim, but true hero and survivor
My worthy friend and artful nurse, the angel.
Who stands on pain and towers over hell
You lead us to a better way of caring
Unafraid to feel, to hear, to cry,
With us and with all mankind.
I'm in good company.

In Just That Way
Joanne Marky Supples

He had this shock of white hair
Pure white, thick clean-looking
Sitting propped up in his bed like the Robert Louis
*   Stevenson poem*
He needed help with his wound dressing
On a weekend when I was on call.
We had never met before.
Even so, he seemed to know me
And looked at me not as a strange but a familiar face.

We talked as I worked on his dressing
Unsure of how this visit would be
I hesitated several times,
Waited for the cues that patients give,
About what he was used to
Or what else he might need on this Saturday morning.
No one else was home.
So I paused to be sure there was nothing more.

He hesitated too, this white-haired man
And I began to think I knew him.
Perhaps from a hospital I had worked in
Had he been a patient there?
No, that wasn't it, he said.
Still, something familiar.

Knowing I would not see him again and having no cause
*   to linger*
I did so all the same.
Reluctantly I said goodbye and wished him well.
He said Goodbye . . . and one more thing.
And then I knew.
He was my grandfather, long dead.
I'm sure it was him all the same.
Because before or since
No one ever called me "Honey Girl"
In just that way.

Radiation Therapy
Shirley A. Mealey

Radiation therapy; warm healing waves of energy
*   coursing through the wounded breast hunting out*
*   cancer cells and killing them*
Radiation therapy; powerful waves of destructive energy
*   coursing through the wounded breast killing cancer cells*
*   and healthy cells*
Radiation therapy; warm healing waves brought by the
*   precise application of technology by caring precise*
*   technicians*
Radiation therapy; destructive waves brought by the
*   precise application of technology by precise technicians*
*   who do not know the wounded breast belongs to a*
*   person whose soul has also been wounded by the*
*   cancerous cells.*

Radiation therapy; which is it?—warm healing waves of energy or powerful waves of destructive energy that kills more healthy cells than necessary—what tips the balance?

Radiation therapy; they say healthy cells have the ability to regenerate while the cancer cells do not—I wonder—I wonder if the healthy cells of a wounded breast of a wounded soul can heal.

Into the fourth week of radiation therapy designed to make it less likely that the cancer cells will not strike that breast again

Into the fourth week for the person who houses the wounded breast to be at the mercy of those whose role is to treat the wounded breast but in doing so wound the soul of the person whose body houses the wounded breast

Into the fourth week—perhaps there is a way for the healing waves of radiation to take charge and heal the wounded breast as the soul begins to heal.

Expendable Notions
Patricia M. Casey

Infant girl without a name
Belonging only to God
Abandoned
Lost
Forgotten.
Perfection describes exterior
Defective, they say, interior
They run; damaged goods.
Still, a heart, a heart that beats . . .
A human soul entwined
within this infinite universe.
Forever left to flutter
Exposed, vulnerable

So alone
We embrace all that is you!
with mature reverence and respect

Human connection: presence
No mother, no father
for earthly comfort
We are here for you
as cruel untimely circumstance
    Pulls . . .   Pulls . . .
       toward the light
       and renewed
       Perfection.

Pain
Suzanne Kusserow

My mind is in my leg.
My head is in my leg.
My world is in my leg.
I cannot talk.
I put up signs:
   KEEP OUT
   NO TRESPASSING
There is nothing here
   but this.

When the morphine kicks in

I can dance the cha cha.
Ride a Persian carpet.
Plant my white leg
in my new-dug zinnia bed
to mock the earth that
once would swallow me.

My world blossoms.

In slow motion
licks of red-hot

blue-white ice dart
  like quick-silver
  minnows
in and out.
I cry—as one does
at the beginnings and
endings of things—
And creep into my leg again.

18

A Brief Tale of Summer

Jennifer B. Averill

PREFACE

What is the creative skein linking the traditional arts of nursing and storytelling? Perhaps it is related to the innate desire to know about the other, both in ourselves and outside of ourselves. The motivation to understand each other and how we relate incites us to creatively explore the range of human experience.

As seekers and as nurses, we engage in focused observation and interaction with people. It is a kind of appraisal or taking in which moves us to inquire, to wonder, to peruse. It is as much an aesthetic, intuitive endeavor as it is empirical, continually emerging as a shared encounter.

At the same time we listen attentively with our ears and our hearts to the stories unfolding before us. We hear not only the

From *Public Health Nursing, 11*(2), April 1994. Reprinted by permission of Blackwell Scientific Publications, Inc.

words and context, but also the sentiments and impressions people express. Joy and sorrow, intrigue and frustration, ritual and ceremony—we take in the total ethos, and we are inevitably touched and changed by it.

We spend time reflecting on the meaning of what we have shared and learned. A kind of quiet analysis then unites the patchwork of senses and intuition within us, yielding a patterned impression which can be expressed in a variety of ways.

In preparing to share the insights we have gained, we realize that empirical expression would limit us to describing, explaining, or predicting what we have accessed through our senses (Carper, 1978; Chinn & Kramer, 1991). It would necessitate the use of facts, models, and theories in order to deduce the significance of our experiences. It would repress the unfettered force of inventive, inductive energy. It would limit the knower to a mere glimpse of the whole.

In the language of Chinn and Kramer (1991), we endeavor instead to creatively *engage* the energies of ourselves and those we seek to understand. In our reflection of experiences, we *interpret* what has occurred in the moment of *experience-action.* We seek to *envision* meaning in the human experience, not only for what has been, but for what it may become. The expression of this innovation comes in the act of writing unique stories and in the art of visual representation. Language and art combine in an attempt to weave the myriad colors of human existence into a tapestry. The knower can sense and intuit much more than the simple facts from such an evocative ethnography. "What is shared in the art/act becomes part of shared understanding in the form of aesthetic knowledge, allowing for appreciation of the experience of the other" (Chinn & Kramer, 1991, p. 11).

Nurses are repeatedly involved in deeply personal interactions with others, often incorporating the enterprises of skilled tasks and information sharing (Benner, 1984; Benner & Wrubel, 1989; Chinn & Kramer, 1991). Thus, the opportunity exists to develop and nurture not only the science of the discipline, but also the art. The inspired expression of narratives and art offers a novel perspective of the shared human experience. Insights and fresh knowledge about phenomena are made possible. Nursing knowledge, in general, can benefit from the authentic incorporation of multi-faceted ways of knowing, exploring, and expressing.

Particular nursing knowledge about migrant farm families is a primary interest of the author. Her concern stems from a long-standing involvement with rural health, as well as from her summer as a migrant education nurse. She combines storytelling and original art in an effort to meaningfully interpret a migrant family's experience in Colorado. (All names of persons are fictitious in the story.) She envisions an enhanced perspective of migrant health, especially as it relates to nursing's informed interest and engagement.

REFERENCES

Benner, P. (1984). *From novice to expert: Excellence and power in clinical nursing practice.* Menlo Park, CA: Addison-Wesley.

Benner, P., & Wrubel, J. (1989). *The primacy of caring: Stress and coping in health and illness.* Menlo Park, CA: Addison-Wesley.

Carper, B. A. (1978). Fundamental patterns of knowing in nursing. *Advances in Nursing Science, 1*(1), 13–23.

Chinn, P. L., & Kramer, M. K. (1991). *Theory and nursing: A systematic approach.* St. Louis: Mosby.

A BRIEF TALE OF SUMMER

Prologue

This is a short story about a migrant family in Colorado. It is not intended to be an in-depth analysis or assessment of the migrant condition. It does not pretend to develop the personalities or characters in depth. Rather, it is a personal vignette of the Rodriguez family. By providing the reader a realistic, narrative glimpse of their lives, the author hopes to enliven a vision of migrant life. The only sources utilized in the preparation of the story are the author's nursing experiences and the work of Littlefield and Stout (1987). Two illustrations are provided by the author to augment and enhance awareness.

Beginning the Journey

It was Manuel and Lucinda in the warm Chihuahua sun that day, loading their few belongings into flour sacks for the long trip north: two cooking pots; a skillet; a bowl, cup, and spoon for each family member; two long wooden spoons for cooking utensils; a ten-foot piece of cotton rope for a clothesline; one change of clothes for Manuel, Lucinda, and each child—Ernesto, Socorra, Josephina, and Miguelito. Manuel and Ernesto each wore a sweat-stained straw hat; Lucinda wore a simple muslin bandana around her head. Two green woolen blankets were folded into place in the front seat of the blue Chevrolet sedan. The family would sleep in the car each night of the journey, sharing the oft-used blankets. They also loaded a metal five-gallon bucket and some homemade soap. It would be the reservoir for bathing and washing clothes over the summer.

Lucinda filled the trunk with ten pounds of flour, a stack of fresh flour tortillas, and a generous bag of fruit given by neighbors and relatives. These items constituted their food supply for the trip to Colorado. It was not abundant, but it was adequate.

Manuel had traded their pesos for all the American dollars he could—$82.50. The money would buy their gasoline and some occasional coffee or pop. It would have to last all the way to Fort Lupton, or they would have to stop along the way and find temporary work. No matter what, they wanted to reach Colorado as soon as possible, to successfully compete for the migrant job openings.

Now they warmly embraced Guadalupe, Lucinda's white-haired mother; her brown, leathery arms and her gnarled hands grasped the family to her breast, and some tears came softly for a few moments. Her own husband, Estevan, had died in the fields eleven years earlier, and she would miss these who shared her blood and her three-room adobe house. But she still had Flavio, Lucinda's brother, who had lost an arm in a farming accident. Her own sisters, Elena and Magdalena, lived next door. She looked around to see other younger people leaving the village for work north of the border. It was planting time in Colorado and other states, and they would all follow the work. It was, after all, a better living than they could manage here.

So into the old Chevy the Rodriguez family climbed. Manuel started it up with a roar, then it quieted somewhat. They headed north as legal aliens, into the morning sun of late May. This car would be their home for the foreseeable future.

The Search

It had taken five days to make this long drive. It could have been three, except for two flat tires and a radiator hose that had to be replaced. At last Fort Lupton shone like a diamond in the distance at midnight. The weary family pulled to the side of the road on the eastern edge of the town, very near one of the fields belonging to the grower they knew. Grateful to have reached their primary destination, they slept without eating that night. As the eastern sky first brightened with the coming dawn, Manuel, Lucinda, and Ernesto stood outside the surplus barracks building, waiting to sign up for summer employment.

Socorra would keep Josephina and Miguelito with her in the car until their parents returned, however long that took. She was twelve this year, and she was quite experienced in caring for her younger siblings, nine and six years old, respectively. Since Ernesto was now fifteen, he could be counted on for a full paycheck for the family.

By noon there were 33 people waiting outside the barracks for word of their hiring. Shortly after one o'clock, a burly man of some fifty years opened the door and stood on the steps. He and his family were settled out now (permanently living in the community year-round), residents of Greeley since 1987. As he gazed at the anxious people before him, he remembered when his own family came to town from Matamoros, Mexico. Then he told them what they came to hear—there was work, but only for thirty souls—no more. They would plant, tend, and harvest the onions, cabbage, and corn for the grower. Then he turned back inside, taking a seat at a rickety wooden table. He signed people up in order of their arrival in front of him. A family of three brothers who had only arrived minutes earlier departed for the next farm, since they were too late to be included here.

Manuel, Lucinda, and Ernesto successfully signed up and smiled to each other. All of the workers were then ordered to begin preparing the fields for planting early the next morning. For now, they were directed to seek what housing they could find among the migrant shacks on the farm's treeless southern perimenter.

Eagerly, Manuel drove his family the six miles from the barracks to the southern fence. The usually dusty road was now more muddy than anything, thanks to last week's late spring snow. Still the old Chevy made it to the edge of the cornfield, and the hungry eyes of the family searched the scattered shacks. Already, all but two were occupied by earlier arrivals, but they found one unoccupied, very near the road (Figure 1).

They had enough tortillas and oranges to last until Sunday, three days away. That would be the one day free, and with their remaining $17.60 they would purchase some pinto beans, more flour, some lard and salt, and maybe some coffee, all in Fort Lupton's only grocery store.

Their home for the summer was modest—plywood and sheet metal enclosing two small rooms. One old stool stood at the doorway; there were no other furnishings. The flooring consisted of

Figure 1. Summer Home for the Rodriquez Family

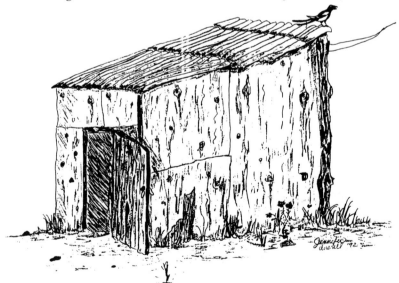

plywood laid over swept, hard-packed earth. A nearby diesel generator supplied electricity to this labor camp. In each shack was one light, a bare bulb, as well as a 1970s vintage electric stove. In the Rodriguez shack, only two of the burners were functional; the oven was not.

Approximately fifty feet from their doorway was a well with a hand pump—the water supply for this cluster of dwellings. Thirty yards south of their hut stood an aging outhouse, again shared with the other dwellers. It had seen its better days, but the weathered structure still had a metal roof and a door; it straddled an irrigation ditch.

Immediately Lucinda drew a bucket of cold water from the pump, and she began to bathe the two younger children. By nightfall, all of them had washed and eaten. Lucinda and Socorra had washed one entire set of clothes for the family, hanging them to dry on a makeshift clothesline inside the shack. This night they slept in the car once again, since it was more comfortable, and it did a better job of keeping them from the late spring wind.

They had made it once again to Colorado, that magnificently beautiful place of snow-capped peaks and fertile plains. Those plains meant employment to them; the mountains insured that enough rain would fall to keep the crops thriving. The summer thunderstorms were legendary, but they took their chances in the weeks between June and September. It was immensely important to family members here and back in Mexico.

The Hanging On

Every morning now but Sunday, Manuel, Lucinda, and Ernesto left before daybreak for the fields. On some days they were able to walk to fields close to their house; other days would find them driving their car the few miles to the appropriate field. They would park alongside the dirt road, then commence hoeing, planting, weeding, thinning, or irrigating the young onions, cabbage, and corn. They worked steadily until noon, then broke half an hour for the lunch they carried with them. They worked on until 6:00 P.M., finally heading for home. The sun beat down, or the thunderstorms brought a squall of rain and wind. Still they persisted, paid by the hour a barely minimum wage every other Saturday. This grower was more generous and reliable than some of the others they knew about in the area. Still there were no bathrooms or running water to drink out in the fields. Workers were obliged to spend their own time traveling back to their shacks if they needed such amenities during working hours. Old Pedro, the foreman, made certain of that. He steadily patrolled and watched the thirty laborers each day, never saying much and occasionally joining in the work himself. It was expected of him by his employer, the grower, despite his advanced years.

Sometimes the hands, arms, and feet of Manuel, Lucinda, and Ernesto broke out in a rash. This was due to the application of pesticides to the fields, sprayed by Pedro on his tractor several evenings a month. They never questioned the rash; it was a customary part of their working lives, regardless of where they labored. It was a necessary, if irritating fact of life.

Meanwhile the migrant summer school recruiter visited one evening their first week there. She signed up Socorra, Josephina, and Miguelito for the summer school session in nearby Fort Lupton. They had to walk a mile to the nearest bus stop for migrant children. They left home at 7:30 each morning, Monday through Friday, returning to their drop-off point around 4:30 P.M. At school each day they received a hot lunch with milk. They attended classes all day, with grades K through 12 all in one building, the local high school. As in all migrant schools, the class sizes were largest in the lower grades, decreasing steadily as the ages of the children advanced. The upper three grades had only a handful of students, since most youngsters in this age group had gone to work in the fields with their parents.

Through the first month of school all the migrant children were screened by two migrant nurses for hearing, vision, scoliosis, hematocrit, and blood pressure. This time, Socorra was found to need glasses. Since the program itself does not purchase the glasses, one of the nurses visited Manuel and Lucinda one evening. She explained the need, asking if they could afford any of the cost of the glasses. The remainder of the cost would be solicited by the nurse from local merchants, on behalf of the migrant children. The

Rodriguez family was able to give her $15.00 toward the cost; the remainder was donated a month later, and Socorra got her glasses.

Another part of school life was appropriate immunization and dental care. Each of the Rodriguez children had numerous caries and gum disease. By the end of August, the visiting dentist had pulled seven teeth and filled 25 cavities among these three children. They were the rule in this group of students, rather than the exception.

In the classes, the bilingual teachers focused on basic skills of reading, writing, simple arithmetic, and an introduction to computers. Several field trips took place over the summer—to interschool sporting events, to a reservoir for a half day of swimming, and to a business in Fort Collins. For these children it was a busy time, a time of some learning and discovery, and a time of physical discomfort because of the dental pain.

It was a time of contrast, as well. By day they read and heard of people, places, and situations entirely foreign to them. Their imaginations were allowed to expand because of their experiences. They became aware of the wondrous technology and varied worlds a used MacIntosh computer could yield. By night they returned to the life known to generations before them, one spare and demanding, offering little save the warmth of the family bond. Sometimes Socorra talked to her mother over the evening chores of meal preparation and clean-up. Lucinda always smiled and encouraged her curious daughter, asking her to share some of her daily experiences.

Manuel and Lucinda had seen neither nurse nor physician in years now. There simply was no provision in the migrant health program funding structure for adult health care. Colorado was one of the few states to offer any kind of health/education program for the children, let alone the workers themselves. One evening in July two nurses and a physician assistant came by their labor camp in a small bus, offering to assess blood pressures and do some general check-ups for the adults. However, Manuel and Lucinda did not avail themselves of the services. They had talked, and they just feared finding a problem for which there was no apparent solution in their lives.

The Departure

It had been a good summer, all things considered. The violent thunderstorms of early summer had spawned two tornadoes in June, both of which drove the frightened workers from the fields and kept them from working two days. Lucinda was sick another day; her head throbbed from the pain of sinusitis, fatigue, and some bad teeth. However, one day of welcome rest out of the sun brought back enough energy to carry on with the harvest. Other than those setbacks, Manuel, Lucinda, and Ernesto worked six days every week. Pedro had previously persuaded the grower that the workers were most productive with one day of rest out of seven.

The first chill of early September brought the final yield of onions and corn (Figure 2). The cabbage had already been gathered, washed, and sent to market. One Wednesday afternoon, Pedro paid the workers their last wages, and then he sent them on their way. The Rodriguez family had saved enough to buy a modest

Figure 2. Manuel and Lucinda Finishing the Corn Harvest

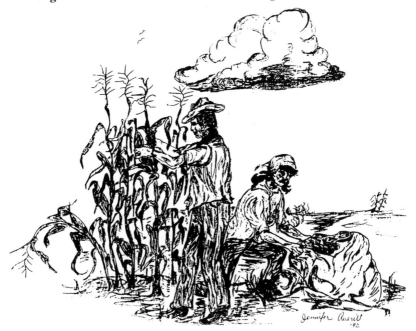

supply of beans, corn, flour, lard, salt, sugar, and coffee. The migrant health clothing/supply bank provided each family member with some much needed attire and even a small Coleman stove. They were quite pleased.

By nightfall they were gone, en route through parts of Oklahoma, Texas, and New Mexico. They might be fortunate enough to find extra work harvesting apples, pecans, and chile in southern New Mexico. They would give it a try, for everything they could earn now would go farther once they got home to Guadalupe and the others.

As they drove through the starlit night on the plains, Manuel and Lucinda began to sing one of their favorite songs. The page turned on another migrant summer, and Lucinda wondered when she should tell Manuel and the others that next summer there would be another member of the family. Together they sang:

Han nacido en mi rancho dos arbolitos,
Dos arbolitos que parecen gemelos,
Y desde mi casita los veo solitos
Bajo el amparo santo y la luz del cielo.
Nunca estan separrados uno del otro
Porque asi quiso Dios que los dos nacieran,
Y con sus mismas ramas se hacen caricias
Como si fueran novios que se quisieran.

The translation:

Two little trees have been born on my ranch,
Two little trees that look like twins
And from my house I see them all alone
Under the holy protection and light from the heavens;
They are never separated, one from the other
Because that is how God wanted for the two
of them to be born,
And with their own branches they caress each other,
As if they were sweethearts who loved each other

Chucho Martinez Gil, ca. 1940.

Epilogue: The Unending Cycle

The Rodriguez family represents a composite of many migrant farm families. They experienced a relatively positive summer, free of severe setbacks or complications which often beset others. They managed to save a sum sufficient to marginally sustain them and their dependents in Mexico until the next growing season. The average annual family income for migrants in Colorado is $6,367. Most of these people have little education and no usual source of health care (Littlefield and Stout, 1987).

As legal aliens working for U.S. growers, they are not entitled to a social security number. Therefore, they have no access to Medicaid or similar services. Only their children receive substantial education and health screening, through the Colorado Migrant Health Program.

With a majority of migrant teenagers leaving school for work in the fields, the future prospects appear gloomy for this population. Few of them graduate from high school, and even fewer ever find a way to attend college. Until the resources of our own society are shared more equitably with these workers, significant improvement for them is probably unlikely.

Meanwhile we shop at supermarkets where gleaming aisles of bountiful produce tempt appetites and pocketbooks. How often do we stop to think how that bounty came to be—grown and nurtured, harvested and washed, ready for our purchase and consumption?

REFERENCES

Littlefield, C. N., & Stout, D. L. (1987). *Access to health care: A survey of Colorado's migrant farm workers.* Denver: Colorado Migrant Health Program.

Index